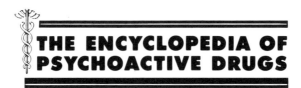

THE ENCYCLOPEDIA OF PSYCHOACTIVE DRUGS

SERIES 1

The Addictive Personality
Alcohol and Alcoholism
Alcohol Customs and Rituals
Alcohol Teenage Drinking
Amphetamines Danger in the Fast Lane
Barbiturates Sleeping Potion or Intoxicant?
Caffeine The Most Popular Stimulant
Cocaine A New Epidemic
Escape from Anxiety and Stress
Flowering Plants Magic in Bloom
Getting Help Treatments for Drug Abuse
Heroin The Street Narcotic
Inhalants The Toxic Fumes

LSD Visions or Nightmares?
Marijuana Its Effects on Mind & Body
Methadone Treatment for Addiction
Mushrooms Psychedelic Fungi
Nicotine An Old-Fashioned Addiction
Over-The-Counter Drugs Harmless or Hazardous?
PCP The Dangerous Angel
Prescription Narcotics The Addictive Painkillers
Quaaludes The Quest for Oblivion
Teenage Depression and Drugs
Treating Mental Illness
Valium The Tranquil Trap

SERIES 2

Bad Trips
Brain Function
Case Histories
Celebrity Drug Use
Designer Drugs
The Downside of Drugs
Drinking, Driving, and Drugs
Drugs and Civilization
Drugs and Crime
Drugs and Diet
Drugs and Disease
Drugs and Emotion
Drugs and Pain
Drugs and Perception
Drugs and Pregnancy
Drugs and Sexual Behavior

Drugs and Sleep
Drugs and Sports
Drugs and the Arts
Drugs and the Brain
Drugs and the Family
Drugs and the Law
Drugs and Women
Drugs of the Future
Drugs Through the Ages
Drug Use Around the World
Legalization A Debate
Mental Disturbances
Nutrition and the Brain
The Origins and Sources of Drugs
Substance Abuse Prevention and Cures
Who Uses Drugs?

DRUGS
&
DISEASE

GENERAL EDITOR
Professor Solomon H. Snyder, M.D.
*Distinguished Service Professor of
Neuroscience, Pharmacology, and Psychiatry at
The Johns Hopkins University School of Medicine*

•

ASSOCIATE EDITOR
Professor Barry L. Jacobs, Ph.D.
*Program in Neuroscience, Department of Psychology,
Princeton University*

•

SENIOR EDITORIAL CONSULTANT
Joann Rodgers
*Deputy Director, Office of Public Affairs at
The Johns Hopkins Medical Institutions*

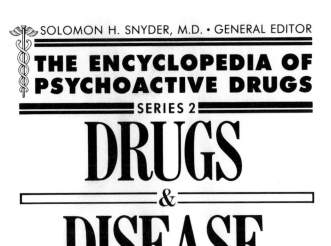

SOLOMON H. SNYDER, M.D. • GENERAL EDITOR

THE ENCYCLOPEDIA OF PSYCHOACTIVE DRUGS

SERIES 2

DRUGS

&

DISEASE

JON ZONDERMAN
LAUREL SHADER M.D.

Rock Valley College
Educational Resources
Center

CHELSEA HOUSE PUBLISHERS
NEW YORK • NEW HAVEN • PHILADELPHIA

EDITOR-IN-CHIEF: Nancy Toff
EXECUTIVE EDITOR: Remmel T. Nunn
MANAGING EDITOR: Karyn Gullen Browne
COPY CHIEF: Perry Scott King
ART DIRECTOR: Giannella Garrett
PICTURE EDITOR: Elizabeth Terhune

STAFF FOR DRUGS AND DISEASE:

SENIOR EDITOR: Jane Larkin Crain
ASSOCIATE EDITOR: Paula Edelson
ASSISTANT EDITOR: Michele A. Merens
DESIGNER: Victoria Tomaselli
COPY EDITORS: Sean Dolan, Gillian Bucky
CAPTIONS: Louise Bloomfield
PICTURE RESEARCH: Diane Moroff, Matthew Miller, Emily Miller
PRODUCTION COORDINATOR: Alma Rodriguez

CREATIVE DIRECTOR: Harold Steinberg

COVER: James Ensor, *Masks and Death,* 1897, Giraudon/Art Resource.

Library of Congress Cataloging-in-Publication Data
Shader, Laurel.
  Drugs & disease.
  (Encyclopedia of psychoactive drugs. Series 2)
  Bibliography: p.
  Includes index.
  1. Substance abuse—Physiological aspects—Juvenile
literature. 2. Chronic diseases—Chemotherapy—Juvenile
literature. I. Zonderman, Jon. II. Title. III. Title: Drugs and
disease. IV. Series. [DNLM: 1. Chronic Disease—drug
therapy—popular works. 2. Drugs—adverse effects—popular
works. 3. Substance Abuse—popular works. 4. Substance Use
Disorders—popular works. WM 270 S524d]
RC564.S49   1987   616'.86   86-33356

ISBN 1-55546-211-1

CONTENTS

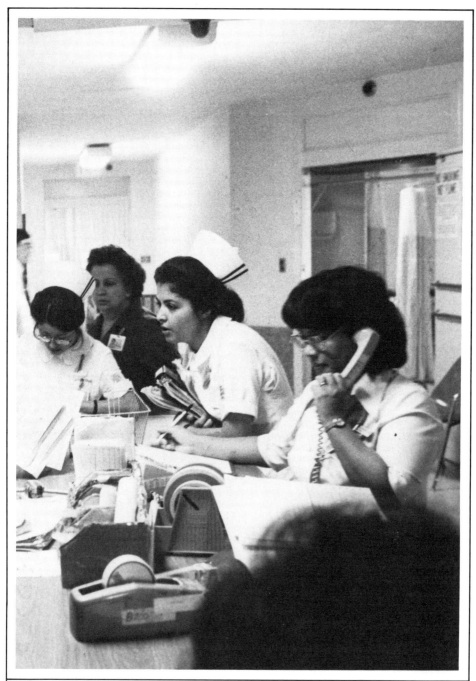

A busy hospital nursing station copes with the demands placed on it each day. Many hospital patients are victims of injuries and diseases associated with the abuse of alcohol, tobacco, and other drugs.

FOREWORD

In the Mainstream
of American Life

One of the legacies of the social upheaval of the 1960s is that psychoactive drugs have become part of the mainstream of American life. Schools, homes, and communities cannot be "drug proofed." There is a demand for drugs — and the supply is plentiful. Social norms have changed and drugs are not only available—they are everywhere.

But where efforts to curtail the supply of drugs and outlaw their use have had tragically limited effects on demand, it may be that education has begun to stem the rising tide of drug abuse among young people and adults alike.

Over the past 25 years, as drugs have become an increasingly routine facet of contemporary life, a great many teenagers have adopted the notion that drug taking was somehow a right or a privilege or a necessity. They have done so, however, without understanding the consequences of drug use during the crucial years of adolescence.

The teenage years are few in the total life cycle, but critical in the maturation process. During these years adolescents face the difficult tasks of discovering their identity, clarifying their sexual roles, asserting their independence, learning to cope with authority, and searching for goals that will give their lives meaning.

Drugs rob adolescents of precious time, stamina, and health. They interrupt critical learning processes, sometimes forever. Teenagers who use drugs are likely to withdraw increasingly into themselves, to "cop out" at just the time when they most need to reach out and experience the world.

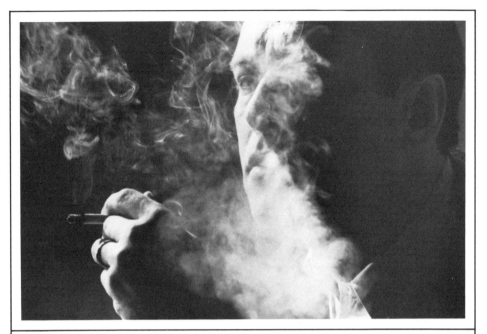

Although the harmful effects of cigarette smoking are well documented, people continue to smoke. Many people who would like to quit smoking are unable to do so because of the power of their addiction.

Fortunately, as a recent Gallup poll shows, young people are beginning to realize this, too. They themselves label drugs their most important problem. In the last few years, moreover, the climate of tolerance and ignorance surrounding drugs has been changing.

Adolescents as well as adults are becoming aware of mounting evidence that every race, ethnic group, and class is vulnerable to drug dependency.

Recent publicity about the cost and failure of drug rehabilitation efforts; dangerous drug use among pilots, air traffic controllers, star athletes, and Hollywood celebrities; and drug-related accidents, suicides, and violent crime have focused the public's attention on the need to wage an all-out war on drug abuse before it seriously undermines the fabric of society itself.

The anti-drug message is getting stronger and there is evidence that the message is beginning to get through to adults and teenagers alike.

The Encyclopedia of Psychoactive Drugs hopes to play a part in the national campaign now underway to educate young people about drugs. Series 1 provides clear and comprehensive discussions of common psychoactive substances, outlines their psychological and physiological effects on the mind and body, explains how they "hook" the user, and separates fact from myth in the complex issue of drug abuse.

Whereas Series 1 focuses on specific drugs, such as nicotine or cocaine, Series 2 confronts a broad range of both social and physiological phenomena. Each volume addresses the ramifications of drug use and abuse on some aspect of human experience: social, familial, cultural, historical, and physical. Separate volumes explore questions about the effects of drugs on brain chemistry and unborn children; the use and abuse of painkillers; the relationship between drugs and sexual behavior, sports, and the arts; drugs and disease; the role of drugs in history; and the sophisticated drugs now being developed in the laboratory that will profoundly change the future.

Each book in the series is fully illustrated and is tailored to the needs and interests of young readers. The more adolescents know about drugs and their role in society, the less likely they are to misuse them.

Joann Rodgers
Senior Editorial Consultant

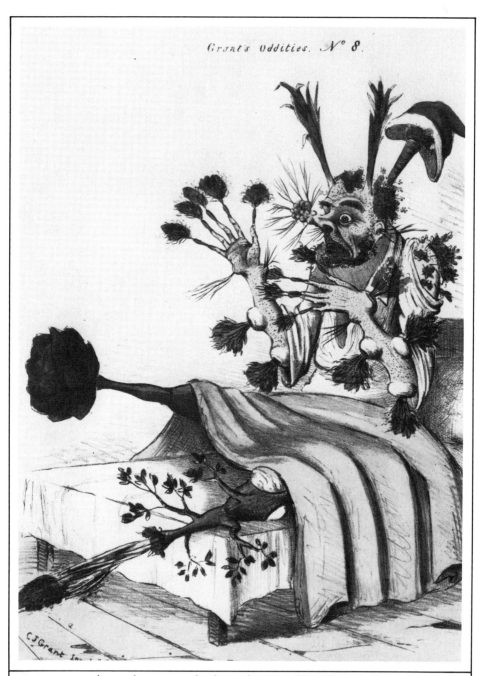

A cartoon takes a humorous look at the possible effects of a "universal vegetable pill." Psychoactive drugs have been associated with magic and wizardry for many centuries. Even in our age of sophisticated medicine, "wonder drugs" are still being sought.

The Gift of Wizardry
Use and Abuse

JACK H. MENDELSON, M.D.
NANCY K. MELLO, PH.D.

Alcohol and Drug Abuse Research Center
Harvard Medical School—McLean Hospital

Dorothy to the Wizard:

"I think you are a very bad man," said Dorothy.

"Oh no, my dear; I'm really a very good man; but I'm a very bad Wizard."

—from THE WIZARD OF OZ

Man is endowed with the gift of wizardry, a talent for discovery and invention. The discovery and invention of substances that change the way we feel and behave are among man's special accomplishments, and, like so many other products of our wizardry, these substances have the capacity to harm as well as to help. Psychoactive drugs can cause profound changes in the chemistry of the brain and other vital organs, and although their legitimate use can relieve pain and cure disease, their abuse leads in a tragic number of cases to destruction.

Consider alcohol — available to all and yet regarded with intense ambivalence from biblical times to the present day. The use of alcoholic beverages dates back to our earliest ancestors. Alcohol use and misuse became associated with the worship of gods and demons. One of the most powerful Greek gods was Dionysus, lord of fruitfulness and god of wine. The Romans adopted Dionysus but changed his name to Bacchus. Festivals and holidays associated with Bacchus celebrated the harvest and the origins of life. Time has blurred the images of the Bacchanalian festival, but the theme of drunkenness as a major part of celebration has survived the pagan gods and remains a familiar part of modern society. The term "Bacchanalian Festival" conveys a more appealing image than "drunken orgy" or "pot party," but whatever the label, drinking alcohol is a form of drug use that results in addiction for millions.

The fact that many millions of other people can use alcohol in moderation does not mitigate the toll this drug takes on society as a whole. According to reliable estimates, one out of every ten Americans develops a serious alcohol-related problem sometime in his or her lifetime. In addition, automobile accidents caused by drunken drivers claim the lives of tens of thousands every year. Many of the victims are gifted young people, just starting out in adult life. Hospital emergency rooms abound with patients seeking help for alcohol-related injuries.

Who is to blame? Can we blame the many manufacturers who produce such an amazing variety of alcoholic beverages? Should we blame the educators who fail to explain the perils of intoxication, or so exaggerate the dangers of drinking that no one could possibly believe them? Are friends to blame — those peers who urge others to "drink more and faster," or the macho types who stress the importance of being able to "hold your liquor"? Casting blame, however, is hardly constructive, and pointing the finger is a fruitless way to deal with the problem. Alcoholism and drug abuse have few culprits but many victims. Accountability begins with each of us, every time we choose to use or misuse an intoxicating substance.

It is ironic that some of man's earliest medicines, derived from natural plant products, are used today to poison and to intoxicate. Relief from pain and suffering is one of society's many continuing goals. Over 3,000 years ago, the Therapeutic Papyrus of Thebes, one of our earliest written records, gave instructions for the use of opium in the treatment of pain. Opium, in the form of its major derivative, morphine, and similar compounds, such as heroin, have also been used by many to induce changes in mood and feeling. Another example of man's misuse of a natural substance is the coca leaf, which for centuries was used by the Indians of Peru to reduce fatigue and hunger. Its modern derivative, cocaine, has important medical use as a local anesthetic. Unfortunately, its increasing abuse in the 1980s clearly has reached epidemic proportions.

The purpose of this series is to explore in depth the psychological and behavioral effects that psychoactive drugs have on the individual, and also, to investigate the ways in which drug use influences the legal, economic, cultural, and even moral aspects of societies. The information presented here (and in other books in this series) is based on many clinical and laboratory studies and other observations by people from diverse walks of life.

Over the centuries, novelists, poets, and dramatists have provided us with many insights into the sometimes seductive but ultimately problematic aspects of alcohol and drug use. Physicians, lawyers, biologists, psychologists, and social scientists have contributed to a better understanding of the causes and consequences of using these substances. The authors in this series have attempted to gather and condense all the latest information about drug use and abuse. They have also described the sometimes wide gaps in our knowledge and have suggested some new ways to answer many difficult questions.

One such question, for example, is how do alcohol and drug problems get started? And what is the best way to treat them when they do? Not too many years ago, alcoholics and drug abusers were regarded as evil, immoral, or both. It is now recognized that these persons suffer from very complicated diseases involving deep psychological and social problems. To understand how the disease begins and progresses, it is necessary to understand the nature of the substance, the behavior of addicts, and the characteristics of the society or culture in which they live.

Although many of the social environments we live in are very similar, some of the most subtle differences can strongly influence our thinking and behavior. Where we live, go to school and work, whom we discuss things with — all influence our opinions about drug use and misuse. Yet we also share certain commonly accepted beliefs that outweigh any differences in our attitudes. The authors in this series have tried to identify and discuss the central, most crucial issues concerning drug use and misuse.

Despite the increasing sophistication of the chemical substances we create in the laboratory, we have a long way to go in our efforts to make these powerful drugs work for us rather than against us.

The volumes in this series address a wide range of timely questions. What influence has drug use had on the arts? Why do so many of today's celebrities and star athletes use drugs, and what is being done to solve this problem? What is the relationship between drugs and crime? What is the physiological basis for the power drugs can hold over us? These are but a few of the issues explored in this far-ranging series.

Educating people about the dangers of drugs can go a long way towards minimizing the desperate consequences of substance abuse for individuals and society as a whole. Luckily, human beings have the resources to solve even the most serious problems that beset them, once they make the commitment to do so. As one keen and sensitive observer, Dr. Lewis Thomas, has said,

> There is nothing at all absurd about the human condition. We matter. It seems to me a good guess, hazarded by a good many people who have thought about it, that we may be engaged in the formation of something like a mind for the life of this planet. If this is so, we are still at the most primitive stage, still fumbling with language and thinking, but infinitely capacitated for the future. Looked at this way, it is remarkable that we've come as far as we have in so short a period, really no time at all as geologists measure time. We are the newest, youngest, and the brightest thing around.

DRUGS

&

DISEASE

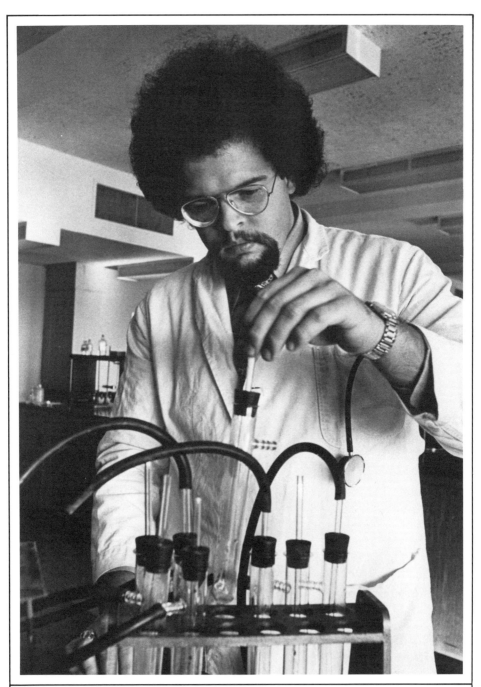

Research has changed perceptions about many drugs once considered harmless. Even nonprescription drugs can have dangerous side effects if they are used improperly or in harmful combinations.

AUTHOR'S PREFACE

The U. S. surgeon general estimates that 350,000 people die each year of diseases caused by or exacerbated by cigarette smoking. These diseases, which include cancer, heart disease, and chronic obstructive pulmonary disease (COPD), may also occur in users or abusers of alcohol, marijuana, and cocaine.

Even over-the-counter drugs available at the corner pharmacy without prescription can complicate or even cause physical ailments if not taken with caution.

This book explores the biological mechanisms by which drugs damage the human body. The first four chapters focus on the four psychoactive drugs most familiar to teenage readers—tobacco, alcohol, marijuana, and cocaine.

Many young people who have experimented with these drugs in the past have not become ill; many of the diseases discussed in this volume occur only in longtime drug users. The body is able to recuperate from many of the ill effects of drug use. For example, the physical condition of many

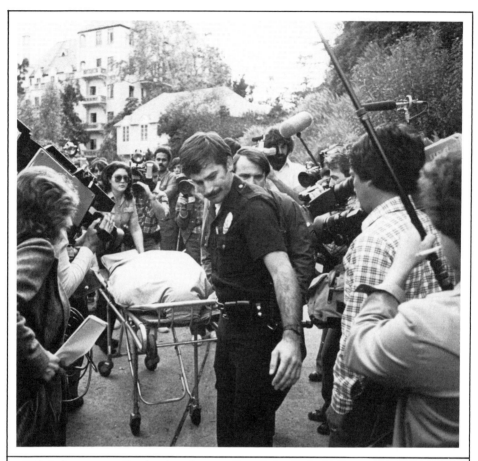

Officials remove the body of comedian John Belushi from a Los Angeles hotel. Belushi, who died of a fatal combination of cocaine and heroin, was plagued by drug problems throughout his life.

longtime drug users, especially smokers, often improves after they have stopped; they may , in time, become almost as healthy as those who have never used the particular drug in the first place.

In other instances, disease and even death can occur rapidly in drug users. Although it was thought for many years that cocaine had few physically harmful effects for "recreational" users, it has been established that the effects of this substance on the heart are so strong that even the first instance of cocaine use can be deadly.

One of the worst effects of drug use in humans is on fetuses and newborn children. Women who use drugs during pregnancy are far more likely to have low-birth-weight children than are women who do not use drugs. Low-birth-weight children are often chronically ill and often have birth defects.

Even when taken as directed, over-the-counter (OTC) drugs can have adverse side effects, especially when taken in conjunction with certain prescription medications or "recreational" drugs. We will investigate those OTCs most often subject to use and abuse. Finally, we will outline some of the detrimental combinations of prescription drugs teenagers might be taking for chronic illnesses and other substances, especially OTC drugs.

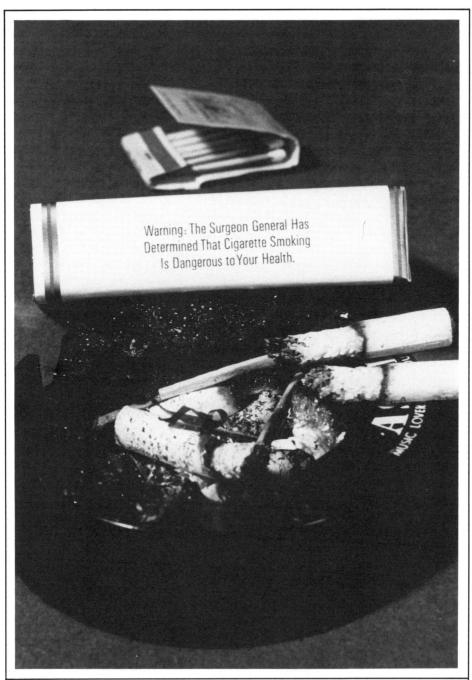

Warning: The Surgeon General Has Determined That Cigarette Smoking Is Dangerous to Your Health.

Since 1964 the American government has required that all cigarette packages display a warning against the hazards of smoking. In 1985 these warnings became stronger and more specific.

CHAPTER 1

TOBACCO

SURGEON GENERAL'S WARNING:
Smoking causes lung cancer,
heart disease, emphysema and may complicate pregnancy.

This warning has been on every package of cigarettes sold in the United States in recent years. All cigarette packages have displayed some type of warning since the mid-1960s.

Millions of Americans, however, continue to smoke cigarettes. Millions more smoke pipes or cigars, and still others chew tobacco or use snuff. Hundreds of thousands of people die each year of tobacco-related illnesses.

An August 1985 report in the prestigious medical journal, *The New England Journal of Medicine,* summarized research into tobacco-related illness. Much of this analysis was done in the late 1970s and early 1980s by the U.S. surgeon general and was released in a continuous stream of reports.

The surgeon general estimated that more than 350,000 deaths each year can be at least partly attributed to cigarette smoking; about 170,000 people die of heart disease, 125,000 from various cancers, and more than 60,000 from long-term obstructive lung diseases such as emphysema and chronic bronchitis.

Each cigarette, it is estimated, shortens a human life by five and one-half minutes. A 25-year-old man who smokes a pack a day can expect, on average, to live four and one-half fewer years than a nonsmoker. A 25-year-old man who smokes two packs a day will cut more than eight years off his life.

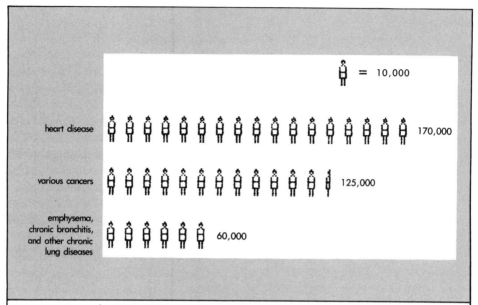

Approximately 350,000 Americans die every year of diseases related to cigarette smoking. Almost half of these deaths are attributable to heart disease; various cancers are responsible for most of the rest.

In the past, when the number of men who smoked was much greater than the number of women who smoked, death from smoking-related illnesses was believed to be an important factor in the difference in life expectancy between men and women. More recent statistics show that although the total amount of cigarette smoking in the American population is decreasing, the proportion of women who smoke is increasing, and smoking-related illnesses and deaths are becoming less and less "men's only" problems.

Health-care costs for smoking-related illness total $16 billion each year. Indirect losses due to lost work, wages, productivity, and premature death cost society another $37 billion each year, according to the best estimates of economists. Each nonsmoker pays $100 per year, in effect, for the medical care of smokers. This money is paid in the form of higher-than-necessary medical insurance premiums and taxes to pay for the health care of smokers covered by Medicare (the health insurance program for Americans over 65 and disabled citizens) and Medicaid (the health insurance program for poor Americans).

The Most Devastating Illness

Although cancer is not the smoking-related illness that kills the most Americans — cardiovascular (heart and circulatory) disease is—it is, in many ways, the most devastating.

Despite all the medical research and the progress in cancer treatment over the past 40 years, cancer that develops in relation to long-term smoking is still almost certainly a death sentence for the smoker.

The survival rate of those diagnosed with many smoking-related cancers, especially lung cancer, is low. (The survival rate for cancer patients is usually defined in terms of the number of people surviving five years after diagnosis.) Treatment of cancer — often disfiguring surgery, radiation therapy, and chemotherapy (treatment with chemicals) — can sometimes prolong a cancer patient's life, but often at great cost in pain and emotional trauma. Quitting smoking can bring the risk of cancer closer to that of nonsmokers over time. (This is discussed in greater detail later in the chapter.)

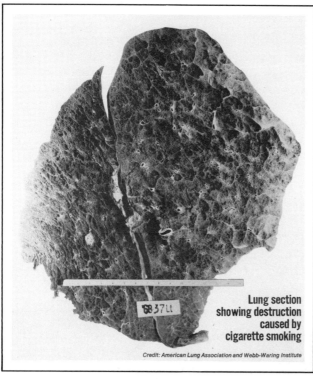

A section of a cancerous lung shows the destruction caused by cigarette smoking. As many as 85% of all lung cancer deaths are related to the consumption of tobacco.

Lung section showing destruction caused by cigarette smoking

Credit: American Lung Association and Webb-Waring Institute

The link between smoking and cancer is not open to question. Some evidence of this connection is provided by epidemiological studies, which are conducted in large populations to determine how much of a certain kind of disease there is in a population and, in the case of a contagious disease, how that disease spreads. Epidemiology was first used to study such contagious diseases as typhoid fever, tuberculosis, and influenza. Since the end of World War II, however, epidemiological practices have been used by doctors and public health researchers to look at statistical evidence of links between illnesses such as cancer and cardiovascular disease and the possible causes of these ailments.

Study after study has shown a direct connection between smoking and cancer. The surgeon general has provided volumes of epidemiological data on smoking and cancer, beginning with the first *Surgeon General's Report on Smoking*, published in 1964, which was the major piece of information used by Congress in its decision to order the health warning on cigarette packages.

Carcinogens and Cigarette Smoke

Another type of evidence linking smoking to cancer is the research that doctors and other scientists have undertaken in recent years to isolate the actual *carcinogens* (cancer-causing agents) in cigarette smoke.

Cigarette smoke, which contains more than three thousand chemicals, is made up of two major parts or phases: a gas (or gaseous phase) and particles (or particulate phase) commonly known as "tar."

Nicotine, the addictive psychoactive component of tobacco products that makes smokers crave and ultimately become dependent on cigarettes, is only one in a long list of carcinogens currently being investigated.

Carcinogens other than nicotine within the particulate phase include the metals nickel and cadmium, and chemicals such as benzopyrene and dibenzanthrene, which can all be isolated from the tar. Carcinogens that exist in the gaseous phase include hydrazine, vinyl chloride, formaldehyde, and nitrogen oxide.

Researchers have been able to relate a few of these chemicals to cancers at particular sites in the body. For the most part, however, it is not entirely clear which components, if

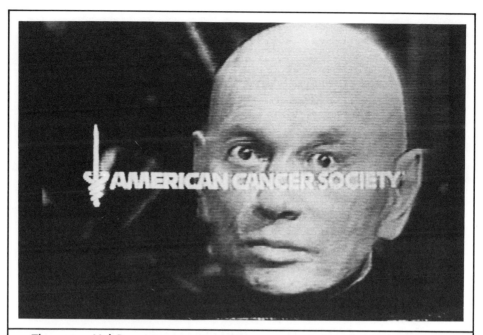

The actor Yul Brynner was one of lung cancer's best known victims. Shortly before he died, Brynner made a television commercial for the American Cancer Society, warning against the dangers of smoking.

any, could be removed from smoke to make tobacco less harmful.

When a person smokes a cigarette, some of the gaseous phase of the smoke is dissolved in the bloodstream and carried to every organ, while some of the particulate phase — the solid matter—is deposited in the lungs.

Some chemicals present in cigarette smoke are also known to be mutagens, or substances that cause mutations, or changes in human DNA. (The nucleic acid DNA, along with RNA, is the basic component of all genetic material. DNA, RNA, and the products they form regulate the division and growth of cells.) Mutations, or abnormalities, in the genetic material can cause errors in cell reproduction and result in cancer.

Lung Cancer

Lung cancer accounts for 25% of all cancer deaths and about 5% of all deaths in the United States. Lung cancer deaths rose from a total of about 18,300 in 1950 to an estimated 131,000 in 1984. Since 80% to 85% of all lung cancer deaths are attributable to smoking, this habit is clearly the leading cause of cancer death in the country.

Although statistics show that more men than women die of lung cancer, increasing numbers of women in the current generations are smoking just as heavily as men, and the difference in the numbers of men and women with lung cancer is becoming smaller. This trend is reflected in the fact that lung cancer is replacing breast cancer as the leading cause of cancer death in women.

The risk of lung cancer for cigar and pipe smokers is far less than for cigarette smokers, but higher than for non-smokers. This does not mean that cigars, pipes, and chewing tobacco are safer than cigarettes. They are related to other types of cancer that are discussed later.

There have been 20% fewer lung cancers among smokers of low-tar and low-nicotine cigarettes, despite research that shows that these people smoke more cigarettes and inhale more deeply on these cigarettes in order to get the same

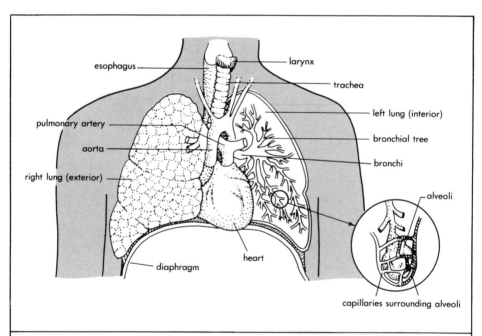

This diagram highlights the major sections of the respiratory system. The various toxins and carcinogens in tobacco smoke can damage this system irreparably, causing cancer or other serious diseases.

daily intake of nicotine, getting at the same time the same daily intake of tar. This statistic suggests that some of the cancer-causing agents in the gaseous phase of smoke can be eliminated through filtering.

The lungs and other tissues of the respiratory tract provide the point of entry for smoke into the bloodstream. Components of smoke are readily absorbed into the lung tissue by way of the 60 to 90 meters of *epithelium* that lines the human airways. Epithelium is a thin layer of cells covering all surfaces outside and inside the body.

Components of smoke reach the sputum, which is made up of the mucus produced by cells lining the bronchial tree (the branched hollow tubing that allows air to pass from the mouth and nose into the lung tissues for distribution of oxygen by the blood to the body's other organs) and old cells shed from this lining. Increased sputum is produced when the bronchial tree is exposed to the irritants in cigarette smoke. Irritation causes coughing, and sputum is often expectorated — brought up. Since it is known that carcinogens, including those contained in cigarette smoke, cause changes in cell structure, examination of the cells in the sputum can reveal the presence of a cancerous tumor that may be too small to see on a chest X ray.

The major methods of early lung cancer detection, therefore, are annual chest X rays, which allow doctors to see abnormal structures in the lungs, and sputum cytology. Cytology is the study of cell structure; abnormalities are detected by examining body tissues and fluids under a microscope. A study of 30,000 male heavy smokers over 45 years old that began in the early 1970s at Johns Hopkins University in Baltimore, the Memorial Sloan-Kettering Cancer Center in New York City, and the Mayo Clinic in Rochester, Minnesota, has shown an increase in survival rate in the group given annual chest X rays and sputum tests in comparison to those for whom tests were suggested but who never received them.

Despite early detection and advancements in the treatment of lung cancer, the five-year survival rate for victims of this disease is only 5% to 8%. This information leads doctors to believe that the only way to control lung cancer is to get people to stop smoking and keep those who have never smoked from starting.

Cancer of the Larynx and Oral Cavity

Each year, 6,000 Americans have their larynx — commonly called the voice box — removed because of cancers strongly associated with the use of tobacco. Although their five-year survival rate is better than 70%, these people live the rest of their lives breathing through a *stoma* — a permanent surgical opening in the windpipe — and speaking with difficulty, often with the aid of an artificial voice box. (Even this type of surgery may not stop people from smoking. The desire for nicotine can be so strong that many patients have been known to continue to smoke through their stomas.)

Other cancers that have a high correlation with smoking are cancers of the tongue, gums, and cheek. These cancers are as prevalent in cigar and pipe smokers as in cigarette smokers, and are also common in users of chewing tobacco and other smokeless tobacco products.

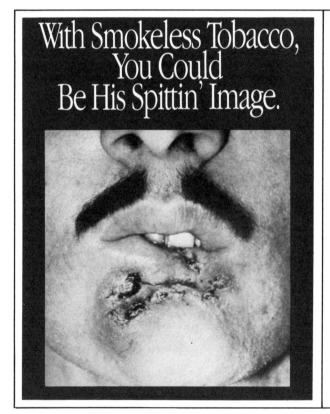

Smokeless tobacco can cause cancer of the tongue, cheek, and gum. In August 1986 the American Cancer Society launched a campaign against this form of tobacco by releasing shocking photographs of actual cancer victims.

An artificial larynx (voice box) permits cancer victims whose larynxes have been removed to speak. Each year approximately 6,000 Americans undergo this operation, most of them because of a cancer contracted through smoking.

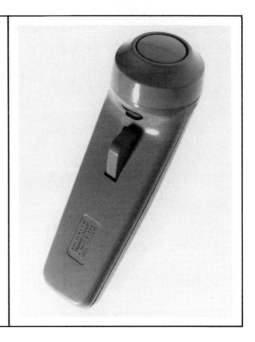

Smokers have also been shown to have more noncancerous mouth diseases than nonsmokers, including gum disease, excessive wear of teeth, discoloration of teeth, and an impaired ability to smell and taste. Cancer of the esophagus — the structure that leads from the mouth to the stomach — is also highly correlated with smoking.

Other Cancers

A number of the carcinogens in tobacco smoke are known to cause bladder cancer, and the incidence of bladder cancer caused by smoking is estimated to be over 25% in women and about 50% in men. Pipe and cigar smokers are less susceptible than cigarette smokers.

A link has also been discovered through epidemiological studies between smoking and cancer of the uterine cervix in women, as well as cancer of the pancreas and kidneys.

Smoking and Cardiovascular Disease

In 1983 the surgeon general reported that "cigarette smoking should be considered the most important known modifiable risk factor for coronary heart disease in the United States."

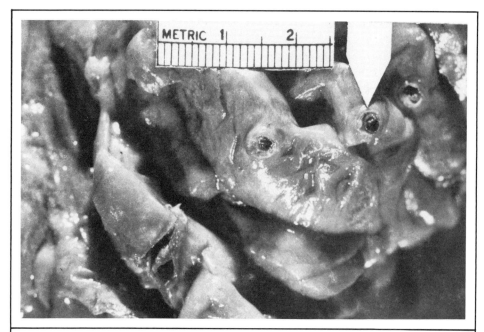

A photograph of a blocked coronary artery. Researchers have theorized that a component of tobacco smoke may cause arteries to narrow, a situation that can result in severe heart disease.

It is estimated that 30% to 40% of the 565,000 deaths from heart disease each year are attributable to smoking.

In addition to being vulnerable to heart disease, smokers are statistically far more likely to have *atherosclerosis* (a buildup of fat on the walls of blood vessels, also known as hardening of the arteries) and other circulatory problems. They are also at greater risk for heart attacks and stroke.

Again, this statistical evidence is based on a large number of epidemiological studies carried out over many years.

The oldest and best-known epidemiological study on heart disease is the so-called Framingham Study, named after the Massachusetts town whose inhabitants doctors have studied since 1948.

More than 170 articles have been published in medical journals by researchers associated with this study, which started out by examining the lifestyle and habits of 5,209 residents between the ages of 30 and 62, almost all of whom were healthy when the study began. Many have since died, and some 4,000 of the children of the original subjects have become a second generation of participants.

The Framingham and other studies have shown that men and women who begin smoking early in life, smoke for long periods of time, and inhale deeply have the greatest statistical risk of developing heart disease.

The Framingham Study was also the first to show a synergy, or a multiplying effect, between smoking and other "risk factors" for heart disease. These risk factors include high blood pressure, high levels of blood cholesterol (a fatty substance found in many rich foods that is associated with the development of atherosclerosis), a variety of genetic characteristics, a lack of exercise, and even stress.

Women smokers who use oral contraceptives encounter an added risk factor. Women who both smoke and use oral contraceptives have a ten times greater chance of dying from coronary artery disease and stroke than do nonsmoking women who do not use oral contraceptives and more than five times the risk of smokers who do not use oral contraceptives. The danger increases for women over 30 who continue to smoke and use oral contraceptives.

Tobacco Glycoprotein

Although much of the evidence linking smoking to cancer is present in the laboratory as well as in epidemiological studies, there is less laboratory evidence to connect smoking to cardiovascular disease.

In early 1986, however, researchers from Cornell University theorized that a chemical in tobacco smoke — tobacco glycoprotein — attaches to the smooth-muscle cells of arteries, causing these cells to grow.

Because the arteries are flexible tubes, an increase in size of the muscle cells in their walls will cause narrowing of the *lumen* — the hollow space inside any tube. This stiffness and narrowing of arteries may impede blood flow to all body tissues, causing such serious problems as *angina* (chest pain from brief episodes of diminished blood flow to the heart), *intermittent claudication* (pain in the legs and often a temporary inability to walk due to episodes of poor blood flow), and *myocardial infarction* (heart attack), which is the death of part of the heart muscle caused by lack of oxygen.

Chronic Obstructive Lung Disease

Chronic obstructive pulmonary (lung) diseases such as emphysema and the more severe forms of bronchitis are characterized by blockage and destruction of the small branches of the air passages in the lungs. They account for 60,000 deaths each year, and they are a painful life sentence for thousands more. There are more than 2 million people alive today with a chronic obstructive pulmonary disease (COPD). Many of them spend their days tethered to oxygen tanks, often too weak to leave their homes or even do daily chores because of the slow continuous deterioration of their lungs.

"Smoker's cough" and brownish, foul-smelling sputum may seem to be merely inconveniences for smokers and those close to them. But these are really only the outward signs of such problems as reduced levels of pulmonary function, which can be the first sign of COPD.

The most common type of COPD is emphysema, an insidious disease that over the course of 10 years or more can destroy enough of a smoker's alveolar sacs — which are gas-exchange chambers in the lungs — to reduce the ability to breathe. After many more years, as many as 40% to 50% of the lungs' 300 million alveolar sacs may be destroyed. A smoker with emphysema can find it so hard to take a breath that it may become impossible to climb a flight of stairs or even walk on level ground.

Respiratory therapists, nurses, and often family and friends must daily pound on the patient's back to clear the lungs of the yellow-brown mucus that clogs the patient's air passages.

The surgeon general has reported that the risk of dying from COPD is 30 times greater for smokers than for nonsmokers. Between 80% and 90% of deaths from these diseases are directly attributable to smoking.

Passive Smoking

A number of epidemiological studies have been undertaken to determine if passive smoking—being present where others are smoking and inhaling this "second-hand smoke" — causes smoking-related diseases in nonsmokers. A number of these studies have involved women married to men who smoke.

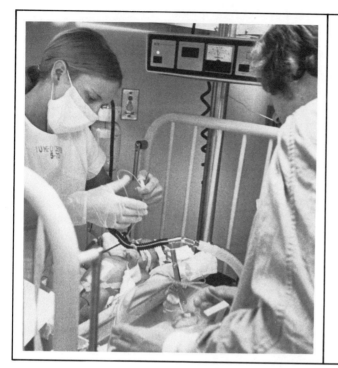

Nurses help a premature infant breathe. Premature birth and abnormally low birth weight are two hazardous consequences of smoking during pregnancy.

There is some evidence of increased heart disease and lung cancer among women in the United States and Japan whose husbands smoke. In addition, both adults and children have often shown decreased pulmonary function when they live in households with smokers.

Other studies have shown that more young children (under two years of age) of parents who smoke are treated by doctors for bronchitis, pneumonia, wheezing, and true asthma than are the children of parents who do not smoke. Middle-ear problems, decreased adult height, and increased risk of sudden infant death have also been reported for children of parents who smoke.

Smoking and Pregnancy

Children born to women who smoke have an average weight of about eight ounces less than children of mothers who do not smoke. These children are also more likely to be characterized as being of low birth weight, defined as a weight at birth of less than approximately five and one-half pounds.

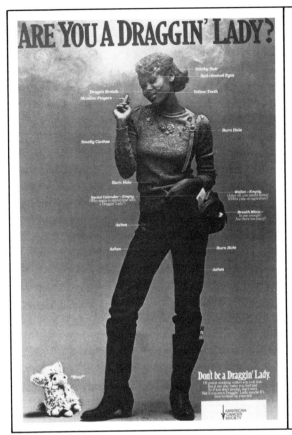

An American Cancer Society poster very cleverly emphasizes the unattractiveness of cigarette smoking.

These children are also more likely to be born prematurely. Premature birth has a direct relationship to higher rates of neonatal (concerning the first 6 weeks after birth) disease and death.

Most of the problems with fetal growth and development may be linked to the carbon monoxide in cigarette smoke. Hemoglobin, a component of red blood cells, is responsible for carrying inhaled oxygen from the lungs to the body's tissues and organs. When the body has used this oxygen it produces carbon dioxide, which is picked up by the hemoglobin and brought back to the lungs, where it is exchanged for more inhaled oxygen. The carbon dioxide leaves the body by exhalation.

Smokers inhale carbon monoxide with oxygen when they smoke. Hemoglobin binds to carbon monoxide very tightly — so tightly that it has a reduced ability to perform oxygen-carbon dioxide exchange.

Fetuses require large amounts of oxygen for adequate growth. The presence of carbon monoxide on the hemoglobin molecules causes decreased oxygen delivery to fetal tissues, poor growth, and the possibility of a low-birthweight baby.

Quitting

Although quitting rarely brings the "reformed" smoker's body back to 100% normal, former smokers can become more healthy over time and live a longer life than they would have had they continued to smoke.

Quitting smoking has been shown to decrease the risk of smoking-related disease and death. People who have stopped smoking for one year reduce their chances of acquiring cardiovascular disease by 50%; this risk reaches the level of a nonsmoker in 10 to 20 years. Similarly, there is about a 40% reduction in risk of lung cancer for former smokers five years after quitting, and the risk reaches the level of a nonsmoker in about 15 years of smoke-free life.

Smoking for any length of time can damage the lungs and other tissues, but kicking the habit may stop the progress of this destruction.

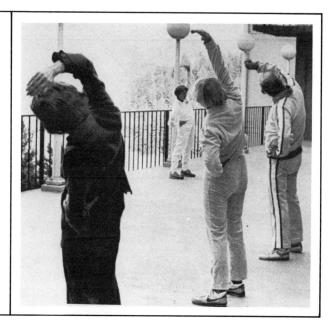

This exercise class is part of a program designed to help participants stop smoking. People who exercise regularly increase their natural energy levels, and may therefore be less dependent on the stimulant properties of nicotine.

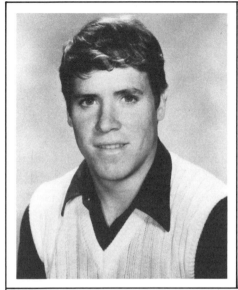 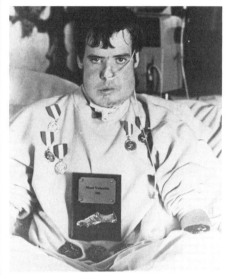

Sean Marsee before and after contracting tongue cancer from using snuff. After Marsee died in 1986, his mother sued the U.S. Tobacco Company for failing to publicize the dangers of smokeless tobacco.

Chewing Tobacco and Snuff

During the late 1970s and early 1980s, television commercials featured popular athletes chewing tobacco and promoting it as a healthy alternative to smoking. Such ads were partially responsible for the sharp increase during that time in the use of snuff and chewing tobacco, especially among young people. Since then, however, studies have linked many cancers of the tongue, gums, and other soft tissues of the mouth to chewing tobacco and "pinching" snuff. In early 1986 President Ronald Reagan signed into law the Comprehensive Smokeless Tobacco Health Education Act, which banned radio and television advertising for chewing tobacco and snuff and required health warnings on smokeless tobacco containers similar to those on cigarette packages.

The American Medical Association, the American Cancer Society, and a number of other health-care organizations have called for a ban on advertising of all tobacco products in all media. It should be noted here that cigarette commercials have been banned on television since the early 1970s, although cigars and pipe tobacco continue to be advertised on television and all tobacco products are promoted in magazines and newspapers and on hundreds of billboards across the country.

Despite the irrefutable medical evidence linking both smoking and chewing tobacco to life-threatening diseases, federal courts in a number of jurisdictions have continued to rule that tobacco companies are not liable for the death and disease related to use of their products. They have ruled that the warning on cigarette packages fulfills the tobacco companies' responsibilities to the consumer.

In June 1986 a federal jury in Oklahoma City voted that the U.S. Tobacco Company was not responsible for the death of Sean Marsee, a 19-year-old with a six-year history of snuff use who died of tongue cancer after three disfiguring operations. Marsee's mother had sued the company for failure to warn her son adequately of the health hazards of snuff.

In short, although advertising for tobacco has been curtailed to some extent, the U.S. government has made it clear that the consumer is responsible for any injury or disease that may result from the use of tobacco products.

———————————◇———————————

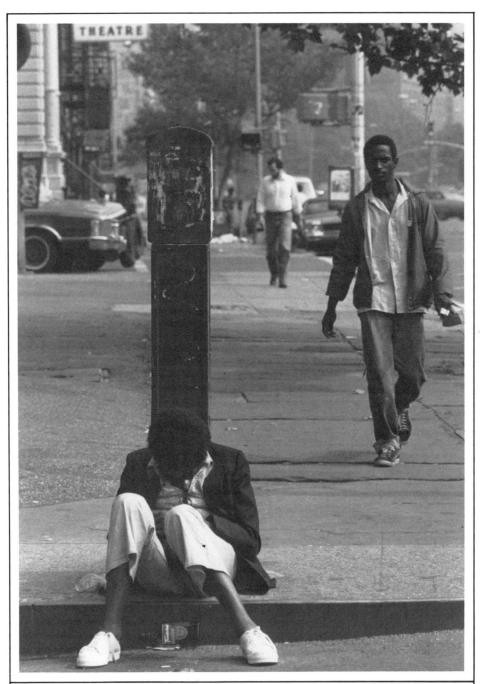

The effects of alcoholism are represented by one of New York City's homeless. Many victims of long-term alcoholism lose their jobs, homes, and families and are in a state of extreme physical decline.

CHAPTER 2

ALCOHOL

Because alcohol is socially accepted and part of a prevalent form of adult relaxation — the cocktail party — it is rarely thought of as the dangerous drug that it is. The dangers of drinking go far beyond the social embarrassments of passing out in public and even extend past the hazards of drunk driving, which can often prove fatal. Quite simply, alcohol is a poison, and researchers have found that it does not take much alcohol to have adverse consequences on the human body.

Although many people think of alcohol-related illness as affecting the "down-and-outers" who drink cheap wine and hang out on street corners, it is a fact that alcoholism and its side effects are present in all social and economic segments of the population.

Alcohol and the Central Nervous System

Most people are familiar with the symptoms of acute intoxication, which include disturbances of perception, speech, balance, and cognition (mental function). Studies concerning drunk driving have repeatedly shown that in the average person, the blood alcohol level achieved by drinking two or three cocktails is sufficient to cause significant impairment in reflexes, judgment of distance and speed, and mental concentration.

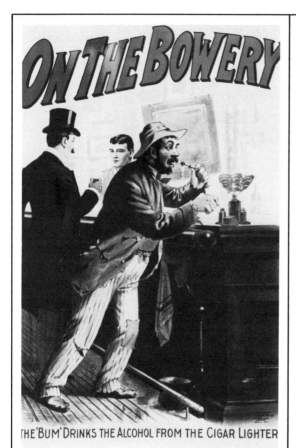

ON THE BOWERY

THE 'BUM' DRINKS THE ALCOHOL FROM THE CIGAR LIGHTER

An 1864 lithograph depicts men from different social classes drinking in a bar. The disease of alcoholism can strike both men and women of all ages and from every walk of life.

Abilities such as concentration, judgment, and coordination are all governed by the central nervous system (the brain and spinal cord), which controls consciousness and mental activities and which is significantly affected by both acute and chronic use of alcohol. Alcohol not only influences these functions of the central nervous system but also affects the passage of chemical messages between neurons.

The central nervous system is composed of thousands of nerve cells that transmit both chemical and electrical messages. Transmission involves passage of these messages across membranes. It is believed that alcohol and its byproducts affect the permeability of these membranes, causing messages either to pass too easily or to be obstructed or garbled. In this way, actions that usually come easily to a person, such as walking in a straight line, cannot be performed properly because messages that govern such activities cannot be transmitted smoothly from the brain to the rest of the body after alcohol has been consumed.

In the chronic alcoholic, the damage to the nervous system is more profound. This impairment is caused by a combination of the direct central nervous system toxicity of alcohol and the nutritional deficiencies that accompany chronic alcoholism. Two classic syndromes seen in chronic alcoholics illustrate this combination of toxicities.

Korsakoff's syndrome, also known as *Korsakoff's psychosis*, is a form of brain damage that most typically occurs as a sequel to chronic alcoholism. It is characterized by extreme confusion and impairment of memory, especially of recent events, while other intellectual functions remain relatively intact. The alcoholic afflicted by this syndrome often compensates for his or her inability to remember current events and facts by making up stories.

According to a recent national survey, an alarming percentage of high school students drink alcohol, often to excess. Teenage chronic drinkers are susceptible to the same physical and emotional problems as adult alcoholics.

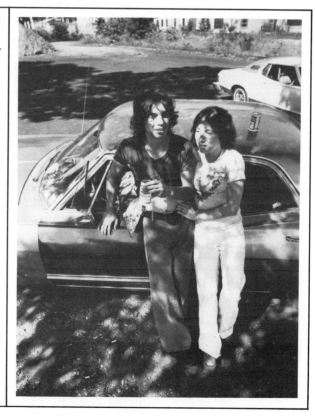

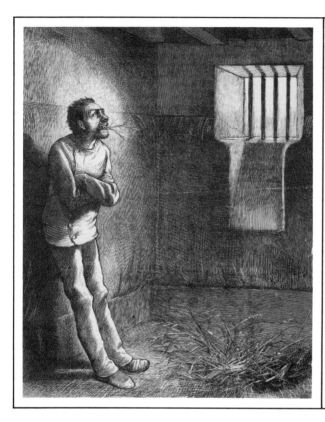

This engraving shows a man undergoing withdrawal from alcohol in the primitive confines of a 19th-century prison. In cases of acute alcoholism, this kind of abrupt withdrawal can be fatal.

Wernicke's syndrome, also known as *Wernicke's encephalopathy*, is the result of thiamine deficiency. Thiamine, one of the B vitamins, is essential for proper function of the central nervous system. Since most chronic alcoholics also suffer from malnutrition, vitamin B is generally lacking in their diets. Wernicke's syndrome is characterized by paralysis of normal eye movements, problems with gait (walking), and disordered thoughts. It can be reversed if thiamine is administered. Wernicke's syndrome is sometimes found in combination with Korsakoff's syndrome, and is often referred to as Wernicke-Korsakoff syndrome.

As is the case with users of narcotics and other addictive drugs, chronic alcoholics who want to stop drinking must withdraw slowly. Sudden stopping of drinking leads to delirium tremens, commonly called "the DTs." Symptoms of the DTs include sweating, tremors, anxiety, hallucinations, and sometimes, if left untreated, seizures and death.

Alcohol and the Liver

Most of the chronic effects of alcohol on the body are related to damage by alcohol to the liver, which is a multipurpose organ of the digestive system. Its responsibilities include biosynthesis, which is the formation of proteins, lipids (fats), and blood clotting factors; detoxification and excretion of toxins such as alcohol, drugs, and poisons, as well as toxic byproducts of metabolism (the process of breaking down a substance into useful or disposable products) such as ammonia; the filtering and disposal of particles and organisms such as bacteria; storage of glycogen (a major source of energy) and vitamins; and formation of bile and bile acids used for digestion and absorption of nutrients. Clearly, the proper functioning of the liver is essential for the proper functioning of the body.

The liver contains most of the enzymes that oxidize (detoxify) alcohol. Because alcohol cannot be stored effectively in the body or eliminated efficiently through the kidneys, lungs, or skin, the burden of removing alcohol from the system rests almost solely with the liver.

The oxidization of alcohol produces *acetaldehyde*, an intermediate metabolite (the product of metabolism) that is in turn oxidized into *acetate* within the liver. Too much acetaldehyde in the body, however, makes it more difficult for the liver to oxidize this still-toxic substance into acetate. This leads to the accumulation of acetaldehyde in the liver, which ultimately causes liver damage.

When most people think of alcohol-related disease they think of cirrhosis of the liver. There are actually three types of hepatic (liver) pathology related to alcohol: alcoholic fatty change, alcoholic hepatitis, and alcoholic cirrhosis.

Alcoholic fatty change, the first stage of liver disease caused by alcohol, is a potentially reversible accumulation of fat in *hepatocytes* (liver cells). It does not have any particular symptoms, but it impairs the ability of the liver to function efficiently. This condition is caused by both an increase in the production of fatty acids and triglycerides (another type of fat) by the liver and a decrease in transport of these products from the liver.

Alcoholic hepatitis is characterized by inflammation and death of hepatocytes. Its symptoms include jaundice — a yellow coloring to the skin and eyes — and a feeling of general ill health. This disease occurs most frequently after a drinking binge — heavy drinking daily over a period of weeks — by an established alcoholic. This type of hepatitis is inflammatory rather than infectious, like hepatitis A and B, which are caused by viruses.

Alcoholic cirrhosis is characterized by replacement of normal liver tissue by fibrous (inflexible) tissue. This condition is analogous to what happens to an orange when it is left in the coldest part of the refrigerator. Parts of the orange survive the cold while other parts become hard and neither look nor taste like an orange. The cirrhotic liver has a drastically reduced capacity to work, because only parts of the liver are available to perform its many essential functions, while large portions have become fibrous.

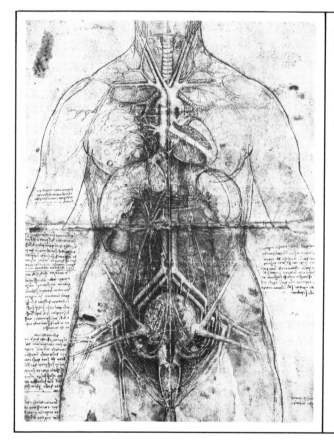

An anatomical study by Leonardo da Vinci. Virtually every part of the human body is susceptible to the long-term effects of alcohol abuse.

Other Medical Consequences of Alcohol

There is virtually no system, region, or organ of the body that is not vulnerable to the toxins in alcohol. The more one drinks, of course, the more serious and long-lasting the consequences.

The Head and Neck

Cancers of the tongue, mouth, pharynx, and esophagus occur more often in alcoholics than in the general population, and numerous studies have shown a marked increase in these cancers for people who both smoke and drink.

Alcohol also irritates the mucous membranes — the most superficial cell layer — in the esophagus, and chronic drinkers have a higher rate of esophagitis — irritation of the esophagus — and Barrett's esophagitis, a precancerous change in the lining of the esophagus — than the general public. Many patients with cirrhosis also develop *esophageal varices* — enlarged, twisted blood vessels in the esophagus caused by back pressure of blood in the fibrous cirrhotic liver — which can rupture and bleed into the intestinal tract, sometimes leading to death from excessive blood loss.

In addition, chronic drinking causes inflammation of the lips and soft tissues of the mouth, as well as enlargement of a salivary gland called the *parotid*. Researchers believe that these effects might be a result not only of the direct tissue damage caused by alcohol, but also of the nutritional deficiency, especially of the B vitamins, that plagues many chronic alcoholics.

The Stomach

Alcohol increases the secretion of gastric acid in the stomach, often injures the stomach's mucous membranes, and is believed by some to promote the formation of gastric ulcers. The combination of aspirin, which is a stomach irritant, and alcohol can cause further damage to the stomach. There is also some evidence linking alcohol consumption with stomach cancer.

The Intestines

Both chronic and short-term excessive drinking can cause structural damage to the small intestine. A single small dose of alcohol has been shown to produce small ulcerative lesions in the *duodenum*, the first division of the small intestine, which is connected to the stomach. These lesions disappear when drinking is stopped.

Vitamin absorption and calcium transport in the intestine have also been shown to be affected by alcohol. In addition, alcohol has a number of adverse effects on lipid metabolism in the small intestine, including decreasing the ability of the intestine to oxidize fatty acids.

The Pancreas

The pancreas, another organ of the digestive system, is affected in many ways by alcohol consumption. Alcoholism and a number of other disorders are associated with inappropriate release of the digestive enzymes produced by the pancreas. This causes breakdown and death of the tissues of the pancreas. The result is *pancreatitis*, an extremely painful disease that can be fatal.

In addition, some studies have shown a high correlation between chronic drinking and cancer of the pancreas.

Alcohol and the Heart

Although the correlation between drinking and heart disease has been known for over a century, it was originally thought to be primarily a result of the malnutrition suffered by so many chronic drinkers.

Recent research, however, has shown a direct link between chronic alcohol consumption and heart disease, especially a condition known as *alcoholic cardiomyopathy*. This progressive (steadily worsening) disease is most often seen in people who have been abusing alcohol for more than 10 years. The symptoms of alcoholic cardiomyopathy are the same as those of congestive heart failure — shortness of breath and fatigue, chest pain, heart palpitations, and bloody sputum, as well as peripheral and pulmonary edema (a leakage of fluid from within blood vessels into the tissues of the arms, legs, face, abdomen, and lungs, causing swelling and restriction of breathing).

Large doses of alcohol have been shown to impair the ability of cardiac (heart) muscle to contract. The heart is a four-chambered muscular pump that collects blood, which has low oxygen content from the veins, pumps it through the right atrium and ventricle into the lungs to be reoxy-

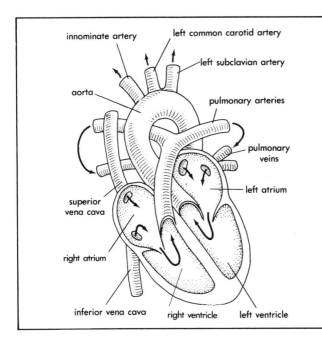

The heart pumps deoxygenated blood to the lungs; there the blood is reoxygenated and pumped to the arteries. The arteries circulate the blood to the organs and muscles of the body. Alcohol can damage cardiac muscle and otherwise disturb the normal functioning of this vital organ.

innominate artery

left common carotid artery

left subclavian artery

aorta

pulmonary arteries

pulmonary veins

left atrium

superior vena cava

right atrium

inferior vena cava

right ventricle

left ventricle

genated, then pumps it through the left atrium and ventricle into arteries, which supply the body with the reoxygenated blood. It is believed that alcohol damages the *mitochondria* — the energy-producing components of cardiac muscle cells. Without energy, the heart pump fails over time, leading to the syndrome of alcoholic cardiomyopathy.

Alcohol has also been shown to induce cardiac arrhythmias, which are disturbances of the normal heart rhythm. Such disordered rhythms can be fatal, particularly in people with underlying heart disease.

Skeletal Muscle

Many chronic drinkers suffer from debilitating muscle fatigue, known as *alcoholic myopathy*. Although more than one-third of alcohol abusers have what doctors term "subclinical," or mild, myopathies, many have a history of severe muscle cramps or weakness and episodes of *myoglobinuria* (dark-colored urine) thought to occur when the body tries to rid itself of myoglobin released by damaged muscle tissue. Acute alcoholic myopathies may include a sudden attack of severe muscle pain or rapidly worsening symptoms of chronic myopathy.

Most episodes of myopathy end soon after a person stops drinking.

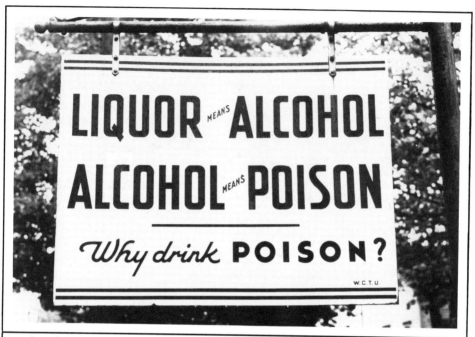

This slogan was posted by the Women's Christian Temperance Union. Although extreme in its position that alcohol use should be completely abolished, this group is correct in identifying alcohol as a toxin.

The Effects of Alcohol on Other Organs

Alcoholics are prone to bacterial lung abscesses caused by aspiration (vomiting and then inhaling stomach contents) while they are intoxicated. Chronic obstructive lung diseases such as emphysema and chronic bronchitis are also common among alcoholics, especially men and particularly those who smoke as well as drink. Heavy drinkers also suffer more often than the general population from pneumococcal pneumonia and tuberculosis, conditions that occur most frequently among malnourished alcoholics. Malnutrition leads to a weakened immune system, making alcoholics susceptible to a variety of infectious diseases.

Alcoholics with liver disease often also have enlarged, fatty kidneys and are more likely than the general population to suffer permanent kidney damage during acute kidney infections. Even alcoholics without liver disease are more likely than the general population to have kidney infections.

In addition, alcoholics often have anemia — a low red blood cell count — caused by deficiencies of iron and B vitamins. Their red blood cells are either abnormally small or abnormally large and are present in unusually small numbers.

There is also some evidence that alcohol directly inhibits the synthesis of *heme* — a part of hemoglobin — in red blood cells. As already noted, hemoglobin is essential for carrying oxygen to the body's organs and tissues.

White blood cells, the components of blood responsible for fighting infection, are also disturbed by alcohol. Both *leukopenia* (a reduced number of white cells) and an impaired ability of white cells to travel to the site of a bacterial infection have been observed in alcoholics.

A Word About Alcohol and Tobacco

Although there is some epidemiological evidence correlating alcohol abuse with cancer, especially of the head and neck — but also of the pancreas, liver, stomach, large intestine,

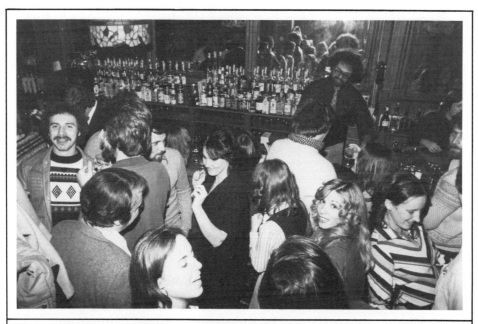

Young people socialize at a Washington, D.C., bar. Because alcohol is socially accepted, relatively cheap, and easily available, it is more widely abused than any illicit drug.

A 45-day-old embryo. Heavy drinking during pregnancy can lead to low birth weight, facial deformities, and defects in the heart and central nervous system.

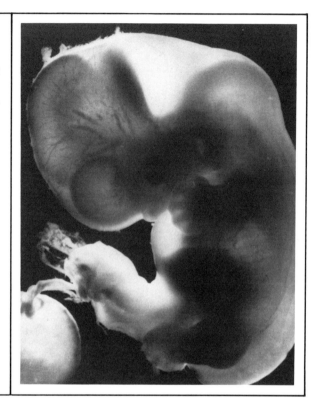

rectum, and even breast — there is no hard evidence as to the mechanism of that association.

Some researchers have theorized that alcohol-induced cellular and enzymatic changes make it easier for cancers to form. Others have speculated that alcohol may act as a solvent to enhance the entry of carcinogens into cells.

Whatever the mechanism, it is striking how many of these cancers are related to the combination of smoking and drinking. Alcohol and tobacco seem to have an additive effect in creating a fertile environment for cancer, especially tumors involving the structures of the head and neck.

Fetal Alcohol Syndrome

Physicians have recognized the effects of maternal alcoholism on the outcome of pregnancy since the time of ancient Greece and Rome. More recently, researchers have described a specific pattern of physical and developmental defects found in children of alcoholic mothers and have labeled this distinct pattern fetal alcohol syndrome, or FAS.

These abnormalities can include problems in the following areas:

• Growth: babies are born short and underweight. They continue to be short and thin as they grow older.

• Facial structure: FAS babies have small heads, small eyes, small mouths and jaws, and may have cleft palates (holes in the roof of the mouth).

• Heart: these children often suffer heart defects; they may be born with holes in the walls separating the two atria and the two ventricles, the four chambers of the heart.

• Central nervous system: brain and spinal cord defects can occur, which can result in mental retardation, developmental delays, sleep disturbances, and hyperactivity.

Fetal alcohol syndrome is seen with alarming frequency in the children of chronic alcoholic mothers. Studies show that ethanol freely crosses the placenta and is directly toxic to the developing fetus. Even moderate drinking by the mother, especially early in pregnancy, may put the fetus at risk.

School daze.

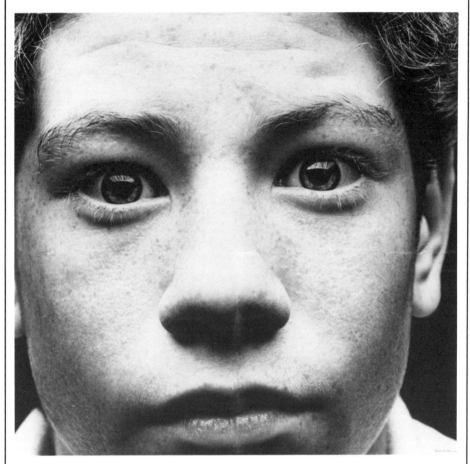

School is tough enough without having to learn through a mind softened with drugs.

So get the education you deserve, and learn how to say no to drugs.

A poster released by the U.S. Department of Health and Human Services is a warning against drug abuse and a reminder that saying no to marijuana and other drugs is a good way to avoid the problem.

Marijuana and Human Reproduction

The two most pronounced effects of marijuana on male reproduction are its effects on sperm cells and their ability to fertilize eggs and its effects on the level of the male hormone testosterone.

The sperm of chronic marijuana smokers have been shown to be relatively few in number, less mobile, and, in some cases, abnormal in structure. Many sperm cells fail to mature. This combination of problems leads to decreased fertility in men who are chronic marijuana smokers. Researchers believe these adverse effects occur at both the local sites, the male gonads (testicles), and at the hypothalamus, which is the central endocrine (hormone-producing) site for the release of hormones associated with reproduction.

The issue of decreased levels of testosterone is more difficult to quantify. Evidence has been contradictory. One of the longest-running controlled studies was conducted over a period of 12 years (1971–83) and involved more than 200

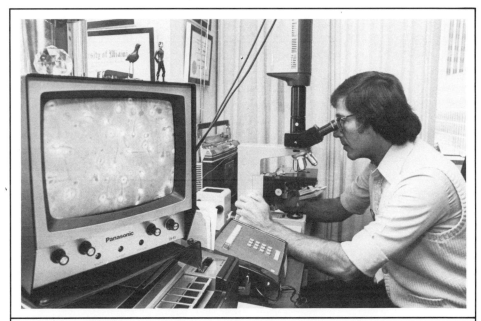

A doctor studies the sperm of an infertile patient. Marijuana interferes with the ability of sperm cells to fertilize eggs; there is also evidence suggesting that it suppresses ovulation.

patients of Harvard's McLean Psychiatric Hospital in Belmont, Massachusetts. Much research on substance abuse takes place in psychiatric hospitals precisely because substance abuse is a complicating factor in many mental health problems.

The McLean study showed no statistically significant difference in plasma (blood) levels of testosterone before and after smoking marijuana, both among "heavy" and "casual" users. Some people who have smoked marijuana heavily during adolescence have been shown to have arrested puberty, suggesting that there may be changes in the hormones that control secondary sexual characteristics.

Jack Mendelson, M.D., and Nancy Mello, Ph.D., who conducted the McLean study, theorized that the finding of decreased testosterone in other studies was influenced by the use of other drugs in addition to marijuana. Alcohol, opiates such as heroin and morphine, and phenothiazines (a class of drugs that includes Thorazine, a medication used to treat psychoses, or mental disturbances) have all been shown to lower testosterone.

Mendelson and Mello are conducting a similar study on female subjects. Their preliminary findings have been consistent with the findings of similar experiments on female mammals, especially monkeys. These results demonstrate that THC suppresses ovulation — the release of an egg cell from the ovary — and the secretion of a number of female hormones necessary for normal reproductive function. The site of interruption of female hormonal activity by THC appears to be at the hypothalamus.

Animal studies have also shown that these hormonal changes affect the offspring of marijuana smokers, especially male offspring. During the first three months of pregnancy, there is some disruption of sexual differentiation of male offspring, meaning that there is incomplete development of male characteristics. Researchers speculate that in humans the endocrine changes in males could cause a delay in puberty, decreased fertility, and possibly impotence.

Marijuana and Fetal Development

Unlike the large amount of research that has been conducted on the effects of alcohol on the fetus, there has been little study of marijuana's impact on fetal development, and there is no well-defined set of physical or developmental characteristics that doctors can associate with the children of marijuana smokers.

Two studies investigating the effects of alcohol on fetal development, however, used marijuana as a variable and did generate some statistical evidence about the adverse effects of marijuana.

A study of 1,690 women and their newborns at Boston City Hospital between 1977 and 1979 showed that, discounting all other variables, the children of mothers who were chronic marijuana users weighed about nine ounces less than the children of mothers who did not use marijuana.

A second study, of 278 women in Denver, did not find marijuana a statistically significant variable in the determination of birth weight; however, marijuana did show up as the sixth most important variable out of 10 entered into the statistical analysis. This means that marijuana is probably one of a number of factors that, when combined, are responsible for low birth weight.

In another study, which involved six infants with the features of fetal alcohol syndrome, including low birth weight, the children's mothers all denied drinking alcohol but all said they smoked cigarettes and also smoked marijuana during pregnancy.

Some infants whose mothers were moderate or heavy marijuana users also showed an abnormally low sensitivity to a light shone directly in their eyes when sleeping. Others showed a higher than normal level of tremulousness, or jitteriness, in their first few days. Still others had an abnormally high pitched cry. Tremors and high-pitched crying are among the symptoms often seen in infants undergoing narcotic withdrawal because of their mothers' use of narcotics during pregnancy.

The relatively small amount of research concerning the effects of the cannabinoids on pregnancy suggests that marijuana can indeed damage the fetus and should not be used during gestation.

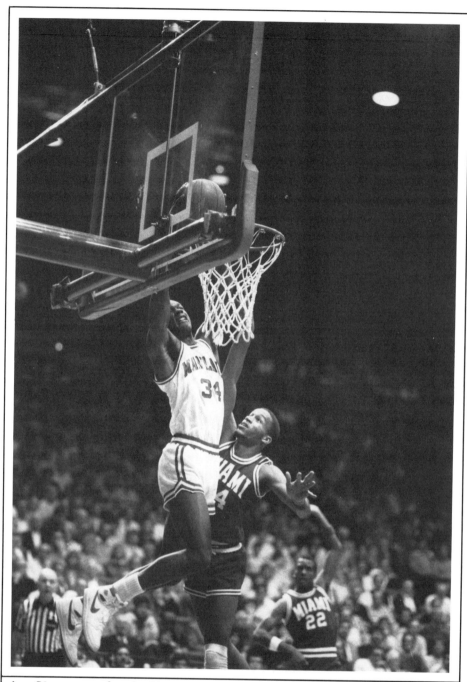

Len Bias scores for the University of Maryland in 1985. Bias's death from a cocaine overdose shocked the nation and vividly dramatized the potentially lethal effects of this "fast track" drug.

CHAPTER 4

COCAINE

In the early morning hours of June 19, 1986, the University of Maryland basketball star Len Bias collapsed in his dormitory room and died. The previous afternoon, Bias had been the first-round draft pick of the Boston Celtics of the National Basketball Association.

The autopsy showed that Bias had been using cocaine.

Eight days later, the night before he was to have been married, Don Rogers, a defensive back with the Cleveland Browns, returned to his mother's home in Sacramento, California, after an all-night bachelor party in his honor. Around 10:30 A.M. he collapsed; by 4:31 P.M., after six hours in a coma, he was dead.

Rogers had also been using cocaine.

The deaths of these two young athletes crystallized feelings throughout the United States that cocaine use was out of hand; and, as the news media and public officials became involved in discussions of cocaine through the summer of 1986, it became clear that cocaine is a far more dangerous and often abused drug than many people had previously thought.

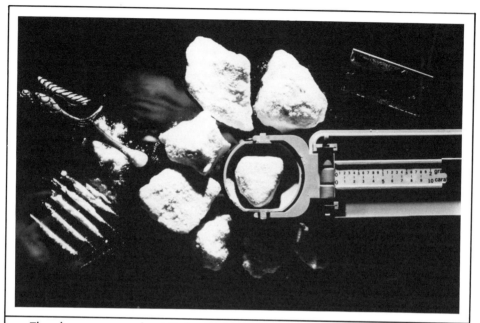

The dangerous and addictive properties of cocaine were unknown for decades. In the 1980s, however, we know that the drug can rule an addict's life long after it has stopped producing pleasurable effects.

What Is Cocaine?

Cocaine is a stimulant that is made from the *Erythroxylon coca* plant, which grows primarily in Central and South America. Although native people in the areas where coca plants are grown chew coca leaves, most users in other areas obtain cocaine, a white powder.

Medically, cocaine is used as a local anesthetic during surgical procedures involving the ear, nose, and mouth, and during bronchoscopic examinations (direct visualization of the bronchial tube through a thin fiber optic scope). In the 19th century and the early part of the 20th century, cocaine was an active ingredient in many "headache powders" and other stimulant "tonics" sold over the counter; it was even an active ingredient in Coca-Cola.

For many years the cocaine obtained by most Americans was diluted, or "cut," with such drugs as amphetamines and caffeine and other substances such as sugar, powdered milk, and baby laxatives. Beginning in the early 1980s, the purity of cocaine in America increased and the price decreased; experts attribute this change in cocaine purity mostly to an increase in production of coca plants by farmers in South America who wish to earn more money on what has become a major cash crop for some nations.

Cocaine is rapidly metabolized in the liver and is eventually excreted in urine. Blood concentration levels peak in about 10 minutes, and cocaine intoxication (the "high") generally lasts between 10 and 30 minutes, depending on the purity, the way it is administered, and the individual's tolerance to the drug.

Cocaine can be taken by oral ingestion, nasal sniffing (often called snorting), intravenous injection, or by freebasing. Freebasing is a dangerous process in which flammable "street cocaine," or cocaine hydrochloride, is mixed with ammonium hydroxide ether. When the solution is heated the ether evaporates, leaving unadulterated freebase cocaine, which is then smoked. Crack, which is crystalized freebase

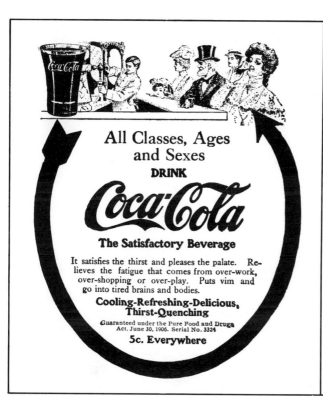

All Classes, Ages and Sexes

DRINK

Coca-Cola

The Satisfactory Beverage

It satisfies the thirst and pleases the palate. Relieves the fatigue that comes from over-work, over-shopping or over-play. Puts vim and go into tired brains and bodies.

Cooling-Refreshing-Delicious, Thirst-Quenching

Guaranteed under the Pure Food and Drugs Act, June 30, 1906. Serial No. 3324

5c. Everywhere

At the time of this early 20th-century advertisement, Coca-Cola contained a large amount of cocaine. Caffeine has long since been substituted and is now the active ingredient in the popular beverage.

cocaine, became a prominent street drug in major U.S. cities by 1985; by the following year its abuse had reached epidemic proportions.

Freebasing crack provides what users described — often in blood-curdling detail on national television newscasts during the summer of 1986 — as the highest highs and the lowest lows. Smoking cocaine introduces the drug into the system faster than other methods, through the lung tissue and immediately into the bloodstream, increasing the danger of acute cocaine reactions.

Until crack became widely available, the majority of cocaine users snorted the drug, which many experts believe was partially responsible for the relative scarcity of acute physical problems associated with cocaine and the misconception that it was a relatively safe, "recreational" drug. It is also thought that because it was a drug of choice for the upper and upper-middle class during its expensive years,

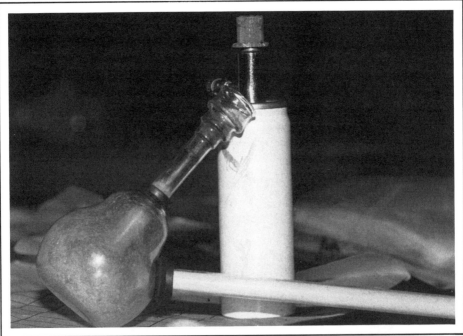

This pipe is used for smoking crack. The use of this highly addictive and crude form of cocaine has reached epidemic proportions among people of all races and social classes during the 1980s.

many medical problems associated with cocaine were able to be hidden. In fact, chronic snorting of cocaine often leads to perforation of the nasal septum (the wall that separates the two nostrils), as well as chronic sore throats, runny noses, and headaches.

The Drug Abuse Warning Network (DAWN) of the National Institute on Drug Abuse reported a 300% increase in the number of cocaine-related emergency room visits between 1976 and 1981, and a 400% increase in cocaine-related deaths in the same period. That number increased again by nearly 100% by 1983.

The increasing awareness of the dangers of cocaine has prompted many users to seek help. According to Mark Gold, M.D., founder of the Cocaine Hot Line (1-800-COCAINE), this organization handled 1.6 million calls from May 1983 to May 1986.

Recent research has also shown cocaine to be a much more highly addictive drug than previously thought. According to animal studies, rats that are allowed to "self-administer" either cocaine or heroin prefer cocaine and will literally eat cocaine until they die. (People who are addicted to cocaine have said they would give up everything and do anything to obtain the substance.) Partly because of their single-mindedness in acquiring cocaine, the experimental animals' general health deteriorates. In people also, chronic use of cocaine has been shown to lead to general physical deterioration, including weight loss, insomnia, anxiety, and other debilitating symptoms.

Cocaine and the Nervous System

Cocaine is a potent substance that exerts its stimulating effects by blocking reuptake (reabsorption) of the neurotransmitter norepinephrine in nerve endings. (Chapter 5 provides a full discussion of the sympathetic response and the autonomic nervous system.) The result is an overload of the sympathetic nervous system and a chemically induced version of the "fight or flight" response.

The cocaine user experiences this sympathetic overload by feeling "high" — euphoric, powerful, and confident. Over time, tolerance occurs, and increasing doses, both in size and frequency, are necessary to achieve the same effect.

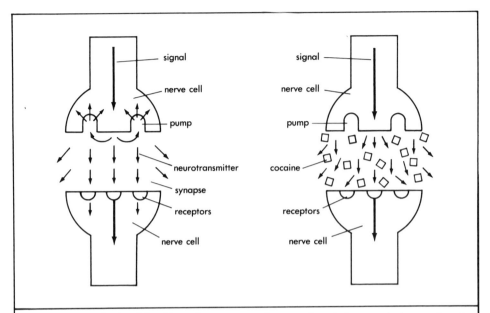

Cocaine works by blocking the return of norepinephrine and dopamine to their cells of origin. This produces a range of feelings from euphoria to anger and depression.

Other aspects of the sympathetic response triggered by cocaine use include increased heart rate, blood pressure, and body temperature, and constriction of blood vessels.

Most of cocaine's effects are far from euphoric. Some users will experience feelings of paranoia, panic, and restlessness. Acute cocaine toxicity, which is similar to that caused by amphetamines, is often characterized by tremors, dizziness, blurred vision, and nervousness.

Babies born to mothers who are heavy cocaine users also experience some of these symptoms, including tremors, fitfulness, sleeplessness, and constant crying.

Cocaine and the Heart and Lungs

At the same time that cocaine forces the heart to work faster, it appears to interfere with the electrical signals from the brain to the heart, making it difficult for the heart to function properly. Even more importantly, cocaine interferes with the electrical conducting system within the heart itself. This accounts for the cardiac arrhythmias that are the major cause of death from cocaine use.

Cocaine increases the pulse rate, respiratory rate, and blood pressure, and cocaine abusers who have convulsions (seizures) may go into respiratory arrest. Many cocaine emergencies involve users who come to emergency rooms with chest pain similar to that of angina pectoris. It may be caused by constriction of the arteries that feed the heart muscle. The chest pain may herald the onset of cardiac arrhythmias.

A number of young cocaine users have been treated for myocardial infarctions (heart attacks); many of these people have none of the other risk factors for heart attack, such as cigarette smoking, drinking, obesity, high blood pressure, or genetic predisposition to heart disease.

The increase of laboratory evidence and statistics on cocaine-related emergencies and deaths indicates in no uncertain terms that cocaine is clearly not the "safe" drug it was once thought to be. As Mark Gold, director of the Cocaine Hot Line, stated on the *McNeil-Lehrer News Hour* shortly after Len Bias's death in 1986, "Cocaine has been field tested by the American public, and it has failed."

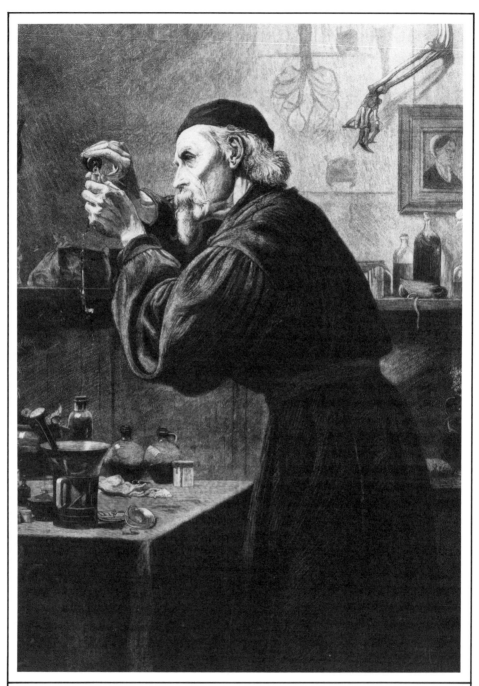

A 15th-century etching depicts a chemist mixing a medicinal remedy. Societies all over the world have used and experimented with healing and mind-altering drugs since the beginning of recorded time.

CHAPTER 5

OVER-THE-COUNTER MEDICATIONS

For decades people have been bombarded by countless potions, lotions, tonics, and pills meant to make them healthier, wiser, more attractive, more energetic, and free of aches and pains. In past centuries, cure-alls were hawked by medicine-show men traveling from town to town. In the late 20th century, over-the-counter (nonprescription) medications are more specialized and are advertised in magazines and newspapers and on radio and television by "real people" who tout their effectiveness.

The most commonly used types of over-the-counter (OTC) medications include pain relievers, appetite suppressants, stimulants, cold and cough preparations, and vitamins.

Pain Relievers

Most OTC pain relievers have as their major component acetaminophen or salicylates. Ibuprofen is the newest OTC pain reliever; until recently it was available only by prescription.

These medications are meant to relieve minor aches and pains. Their manufacturers encourage users to seek medical attention if the discomfort lasts more than a day or two.

Although these medications are likely to be effective if taken as directed, all have the potential for significant toxicity if abused.

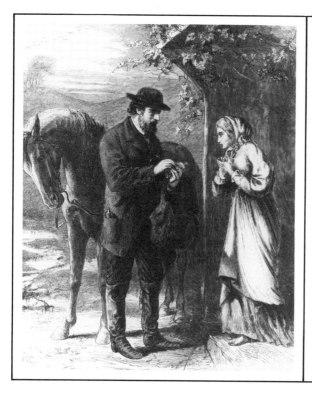

The woman in this 1869 engraving is receiving medicine from a country doctor. We tend to laugh at the "snake-oil salesmen" of old, but in the 1980s the average American household stocks 17 different over-the-counter products.

Acetaminophen

Acetaminophen preparations (such as Tylenol, Tempra, and Panadol) are meant to be used for the relief of pain and fever. Acetaminophen is also a component of many combination drugs (medications that include more than one active ingredient) used to alleviate cold symptoms.

Accidental overdose most often occurs in children under six, who are attracted to the bright color and relatively good taste of these drugs. Older children, teenagers, and adults who take overdoses of acetaminophen as a suicide gesture usually do not realize just how highly toxic a drug it is when taken in large amounts.

Acetaminophen is readily absorbed into the bloodstream by the intestines and is carried to the liver for further metabolism. Small doses are easily handled by a normal liver. In large doses, particularly in people older than six, the drug can damage the liver. Some studies suggest that large doses of acetaminophen can cause irreversible liver damage.

Additionally, people who take overdoses of this medication often combine acetaminophen with such drugs as alcohol, a combination that is extremely dangerous to the function of the liver and can be fatal.

Salicylates

Acetylsalicylic acid (aspirin) was the first widely used OTC drug for the relief of pain and fever and is among the drugs of choice for arthritis.

One of the common side effects of aspirin and aspirin-containing compounds is a decrease in blood clotting. This side effect can be beneficial for patients who have artificial heart valves or shunts (tubes used in bypass operations), because it helps prevent the formation of blood clots, which can restrict the flow of blood and impede the heart's pumping action. These clots can be carried by the bloodstream into the brain, causing strokes.

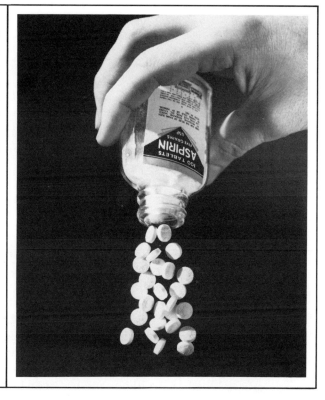

Although aspirin, which is the most widely used drug in the United States, is relatively safe if taken in proper doses, abuse of this OTC substance can cause nausea, convulsions, and even death.

Increased bleeding or decreased clotting caused by aspirin is dangerous for people with underlying diseases such as hemophilia (an inherited blood disease marked by severe, sometimes spontaneous bleeding), in which clotting is already impaired, or colitis, in which there may be chronic blood loss from ulcerations in the large intestine. Aspirin consumption has also been linked to the formation of gastric ulcers.

In recent years there has been an association between the treatment of chicken pox and flu-like illnesses with aspirin and the subsequent development of Reye's syndrome in children under 18. At this point, the cause of Reye's syndrome is a medical mystery, and researchers do not understand how it is linked with aspirin. The disease is characterized by changes in mental status ranging from lethargy to coma, as well as multiple-organ failure. Some children recover completely, whereas others are left with significant brain damage.

Aspirin poisoning, also known as salicylism, can be acute (from an overdose) or chronic (from therapeutic use over a long period). The first symptoms of salicylism are those of central nervous system stimulation and include vomiting, rapid breathing, hyperactivity, increased body temperature, and seizures. The second phase is characterized by central nervous system depression, which causes lethargy and respiratory failure.

Symptoms of chronic salicylism develop over a long period and are reversed when the aspirin is discontinued or the dose lowered. Acute ingestions (overdoses) are treated by emptying the stomach and correcting blood-chemistry abnormalities.

Ibuprofen

Ibuprofen belongs to a class of drugs known as nonsteroidal anti-inflammatory agents. These drugs are used to control pain and decrease inflammation. They also have some action against fever. Recently, ibuprofen has become available over the counter under such brand names as Advil and Nuprin.

The principal side effects of ibuprofen include nausea, abdominal pain, dizziness, and rash. People who are sensitive or allergic to aspirin should not take this medication because it may cause the same allergic symptoms. It may also exacerbate bleeding problems and has been known to cause acute kidney failure in people with kidney disease. Overdose is treated in the same way as aspirin overdose.

Stimulants

Many OTC drugs contain substances that stimulate the nervous system, making the user feel alert and active. In the 19th and early 20th centuries, many preparations containing amphetamines were readily available. They were originally used as nasal decongestants, but when their common side effects — increased alertness and decreased appetite — became known, their popularity increased.

In recent years strict regulations have been developed regarding the use and availability of amphetamines. Drugs with similar effects are now readily available, however, and their use is widespread.

In order to understand clearly the effects of stimulants and related drugs, it is necessary to understand the function of the autonomic nervous system.

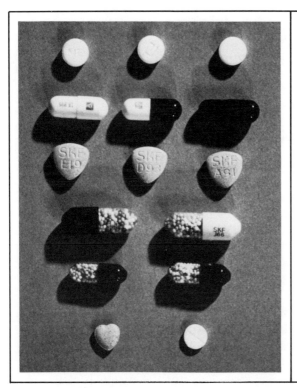

Amphetamines were prescribed frequently for obesity in the 1950s. In the 1980s many people take OTC substances containing amphetamine-like compounds to control their appetites. Symptoms of stimulant abuse include anxiety, tremors, and insomnia.

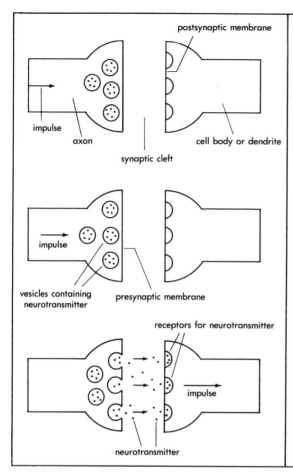

Neurotransmitters convey electrical impulses by crossing the synapse (gap) between neurons. Drugs can enhance or inhibit their functions. Some OTC drugs stimulate the sympathetic nervous system by imitating or prolonging the effects of the neurotransmitters that govern it.

The Autonomic Nervous System

The autonomic nervous system is the part of the nervous system that controls the involuntary functions of organs, glands, and blood vessels. The parasympathetic division of the autonomic nervous system is responsible for the maintenance of *homeostasis* — the balance of normal body functions — whereas the sympathetic division is responsible for the "fight or flight" response to stress. Both divisions are present in most organs, glands, and blood vessels, and are activated as needed.

Information is passed throughout the nervous system by electrical impulses, which are transported from nerve to nerve by chemicals called neurotransmitters. Neurotransmitters are like ships sailing between ports separated by a channel, known as the synapse. The port of origin is the presynaptic membrane; the port of call the postsynaptic membrane. Electrical energy reaches the presynaptic membrane, neurotransmitters are released into the synapse, and they travel to the receptor sites on the postsynaptic membrane. This chemical connection allows for the transmission of the electrical impulse down the chain of nerve cells until the message reaches its target.

When the parasympathetic division is activated, the body is in a relaxed state. The heart rate is at its baseline, or normal rate, digestion is at its peak, and the liver is forming and storing energy molecules for later use. The small airways are constricted and secreting mucus. The pupils of the eyes are also constricted, and the eyes are adjusted for near vision. The mucous membranes of the mouth and nose are moist, and perspiration is minimal.

When the sympathetic division is activated, the body functions necessary for fight or flight come into play. The heart rate increases, and blood flows to the skeletal muscles (those in the arms, legs, and trunk) rather than the gastrointestinal tract. Consequently, digestion slows. The liver breaks down its stored energy molecules to handle stress. The small airways dilate and secretions decrease for better ventilation. The pupils of the eyes dilate and the eyes adjust for distant vision. The mouth and nose become dry, and profuse sweating may occur.

Neurotransmitters and the Nervous System

Acetylcholine is the neurotransmitter that ferries messages between the nerve cells of the parasympathetic nervous system. Drugs that interfere with this neurotransmitter are called anticholinergics. In the presence of anticholinergics the parasympathetic nervous system is inhibited, leading to overactivity of the sympathetic nervous system. Anticholinergics are not found in OTC preparations. Instead, they are administered in specific circumstances, by prescription only.

Epinephrine and norepinephrine are the neurotransmitters that activate the sympathetic nervous system. Drugs that either mimic these neurotransmitters or prolong their action are called sympathomimetics. Such drugs are often found in over-the-counter preparations, such as the decongestants (drugs that reduce nasal congestion) Neo-Synephrine, Triaminic Cough Syrup, and Actifed.

77

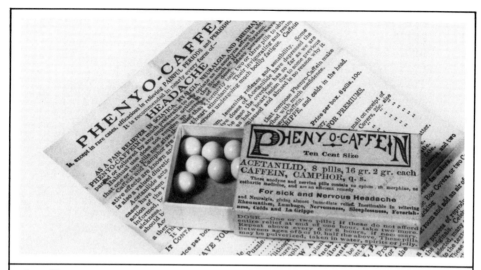

A caffeine preparation from the early 20th century. Many students in the 1980s use such substances to help them study through the night.

Caffeine

The most available and best known OTC stimulant today is caffeine. It is found in coffee, tea, cocoa, and many carbonated beverages. Caffeine is also available in pure form. It is used by some physicians to stimulate spontaneous breathing in premature infants. The OTC forms of pure caffeine include No-Doz Fast Acting Keep Alert Tablets and Vivarin Stimulant Tablets, popular among high-school and college students, who use them to stay awake for studying and other activities.

Caffeine dependence is a common problem. Dependence is an adaptation of the body to the continued presence of a drug. If use of the drug is discontinued, withdrawal symptoms occur. In the case of caffeine dependence, withdrawal symptoms may include anxiety, irritability, and severe headaches. The syndrome of caffeinism (chronic overuse of caffeine, usually in the form of coffee) is characterized by irritability, insomnia, palpitations, and gastric upset. Acute caffeine overdose is characterized by tachycardia (sustained rapid heart rate), extrasystoles (occasional extra heartbeats), urinary frequency, nausea, vomiting, tinnitus (ringing in the ears), tremors, and seizures, all effects of overloading the sympathetic nervous system.

Cold and Cough Preparations

Dozens of OTC products are available for the treatment of colds and coughs. Some are billed as decongestants, others as antihistamines, antitussives, or expectorants (see below). There are also OTC asthma medications available that some people may confuse with cold and cough medications. Most of these drugs are prepared from some combination of a handful of active ingredients. The most popular components include:

Phenylpropanolamine and **pseudoephedrine,** sympathomimetics (drugs that produce effects resembling those resulting from stimulation of the sympathetic nervous system) that treat runny nose by constricting small blood vessels.

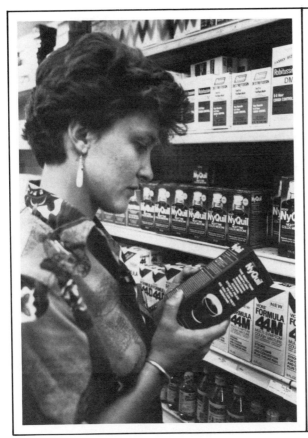

A shopper carefully reads the label on a well-known OTC preparation. Many consumers mistakenly assume that because a drug is readily available they need not question its safety. In fact, OTC drugs can be dangerous, particularly if taken in combination with other medications or alcohol.

Chlorpheniramine maleate, an antihistamine that stops runny nose and red eyes by inhibiting the release of histamine.

Dextromethorphan and **guaifenesin,** an antitussive (cough suppressant) and an expectorant (promotor of sputum-producing cough), respectively.

These drugs also contain varying amounts and combinations of the following components: analgesics (pain relievers) and antipyretics (fever reducers, such as aspirin and acetaminophen), aromatic decongestants (menthol, peppermint oil, and others), and alcohol.

Most upper respiratory infections (coughs and colds) are brief in duration. OTC products will not cure a cold or decrease the duration of symptoms, but they may lessen the severity of the symptoms. Symptoms of allergies such as hay fever, which are similar to those of the common cold, are generally helped or relieved by preparations that include an antihistamine.

Another common symptom of mild respiratory tract infection is increased secretions by the bronchial tree. Expectoration — coughing up — of these secretions helps the body clear itself of the infection and the infecting organism (usually a virus). For that reason it is generally not advisable to use medications that contain cough suppressants.

Side effects of sympathomimetics have already been discussed; side effects of antihistamines include increased heart rate, restlessness or, conversely, drowsiness, and dry mouth and nose. Overdoses can cause seizures.

Dextromethorphan may produce constipation. Guaifenesin is said to be free of side effects. It is important to note that many cold and cough preparations in liquid form contain substantial amounts of alcohol; people who drink cough syrup to get drunk will not only experience the effects of the alcohol but also those of an overdose of sympathomimetics and aspirin or acetaminophen.

When used intelligently, most OTC drugs are safe, and many are effective. It is essential to read the list of indications and ingredients and to use these drugs only as directed. For example, because cold and cough preparations contain sympathomimetic components, which work against antihypertensives (drugs that decrease blood pressure) and antidepressants (drugs that relieve symptoms of depression) and multiply the effects of asthma medications, they should never be combined with these three types of drugs. It is also unwise to use cough and cold medications in the presence of high blood pressure, heart disease, insulin-dependent diabetes, thyroid disease, or glaucoma.

Appetite Suppressants

Most anorexiants (appetite suppressants, diet aids, and weight-loss pills) have the same basic components as cold and cough remedies. As discussed in the section on stimulants, one of the major side effects of the sympathomimetics is loss of appetite, with or without nausea and vomiting.

In the fight-or-flight response, most of the body's blood supply, and therefore most of the body's energy, is directed toward those organs and systems needed for minute-to-minute survival in acute stress. Only the minimum required

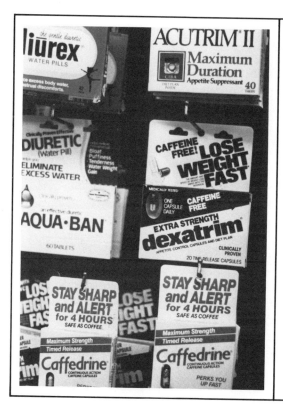

Appetite suppressants are not only ineffective but unsafe if taken in higher than recommended doses. In addition, statistics show that any weight loss achieved is unlikely to last when the pills are discontinued.

amount of energy is supplied to the digestive tract. The result is a lack of appetite, often accompanied by gastric upset.

Two common OTC appetite suppressants, Acutrim and Dexatrim, contain phenylpropanolamine (PPA) as their active ingredient. They are available in sustained-release preparations, which are active for 12 to 16 hours. In the past, many of these preparations also contained caffeine, which increases the stimulant effects of PPA. This combination drug had been widely abused, especially by adolescents. Even with the removal of caffeine from the drugs, the PPA-only drugs, when mixed with the caffeine from soft drinks, still provide adolescents with a "legal" high.

The effectiveness of appetite suppressants in weight loss is questionable. These drugs do reduce the desire to eat, giving many users the idea that they can satisfy what little hunger they have by eating junk food rather than a smaller balanced diet. It is suggested that they be used for no longer than three months; people who do not develop better eating habits while on the drug usually regain most of the lost weight when the drug is discontinued.

Side effects of the appetite suppressants are the same as those of cold and cough preparations. These effects can be severe and even dangerous for people who take more than the suggested dose with the thought that more medication will increase the rate of weight loss.

Vitamins and Related Substances

Vitamins and other substances known as elements or minerals are essential for proper body function. Under normal conditions the recommended daily allowances of vitamins and minerals can be met by a balanced diet that contains representatives from the four basic food groups: dairy products, meats, fruits and vegetables, and grains.

There is a great deal of mythology surrounding vitamins. The concept that megadoses of various vitamins and minerals will cure cancer and make one bigger, stronger, smarter, and more masculine or feminine has been popularized over many years and has been almost impossible to disprove.

The multivitamins that so many Americans take daily probably have very little real effect on their general health and well-being in the presence of a balanced diet. But for

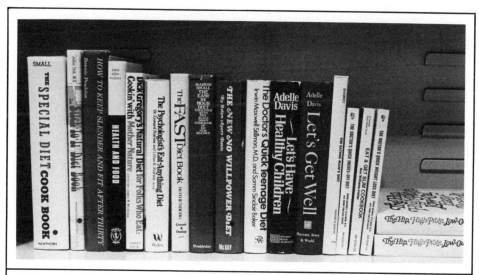

Eating habits that produce weight loss by natural means are far more reliable than appetite suppressants. Countless books are published every year that offer advice on how to maintain a healthy diet.

children and adults who, for reasons of economics or geography are unable to eat regular balanced meals, vitamin supplements may be helpful. A wide variety of conditions, including pregnancy, severe burns, and many inherited or acquired diseases affect or are affected by proper nutrition and may require dietary supplementation or restriction.

Diseases such as scurvy and rickets are caused by vitamin deficiencies. At the same time, overuse or abuse of some vitamins and minerals can have severe health consequences.

Vitamin A

Vitamin A (retinol) is found in leafy green and yellow vegetables, liver, egg yolks, butter, and cream. It is added to most margarine and some bread and sugar. Vitamin A is necessary for integrity of the skin and for proper vision, including light/dark differentiation and color vision.

Excessive intake of vitamin A can cause severe headaches and vomiting, sometimes with increased intracranial pressure that mimics the pressure of a brain tumor, known as *pseudotumor cerebri*. Peeling of the skin and thickening of the bones can also occur.

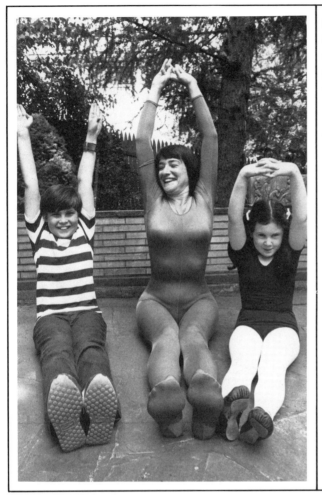

Exercise is essential for both mind and body. Studies show that people who exercise regularly take far fewer OTC products than those who do not.

Vitamin D

Vitamin D occurs in two major forms, and is found in fortified milk, liver, butter, and egg yolks. It is also formed in the skin during exposure to sunlight; this is actually the major source of vitamin D for most people. It is necessary for the absorption of calcium and phosphorus, substances essential for the proper formation of bones.

Excessive intake of vitamin D causes increased absorption of calcium by the intestines and the deposit of calcium in various organs. Calcium deposits in the kidneys can lead to irreversible kidney failure.

Iron

Iron is one of 15 essential trace elements — metals and other related substances present in small amounts in the body. It is found in most nondairy foods. Unfortunately, less than 20% of ingested iron is actually absorbed under ideal conditions. Iron is essential to the formation of hemoglobin in red blood cells, which carry oxygen from the lungs to the body (see Chapter 1).

Iron supplements are often necessary medications for pregnant women, people with chronic blood loss, and people suffering from anemia caused by iron deficiencies. Occasionally, iron supplements are also recommended for breast-fed infants. Iron supplements most frequently take the form of OTC tablets or liquids.

Iron poisoning is seen most commonly in children who accidentally eat large numbers of iron tablets or multivitamins with iron at a single sitting. Initially, iron overdose causes vomiting, diarrhea, abdominal pain, and gastrointestinal bleeding. This is followed by acute circulatory collapse and shock; death may occur from bleeding and heart failure.

OTCs are usually safe if they are taken at recommended doses, for the particular symptoms they are intended to relieve, and with attention to any restrictions stated by the manufacturer. These drugs, however, have the same potential for misuse and abuse as alcohol, tobacco, marijuana and other psychoactive drugs. In fact, an overdose of many kinds of OTC drugs can be just as dangerous — and deadly — as any other drug overdose.

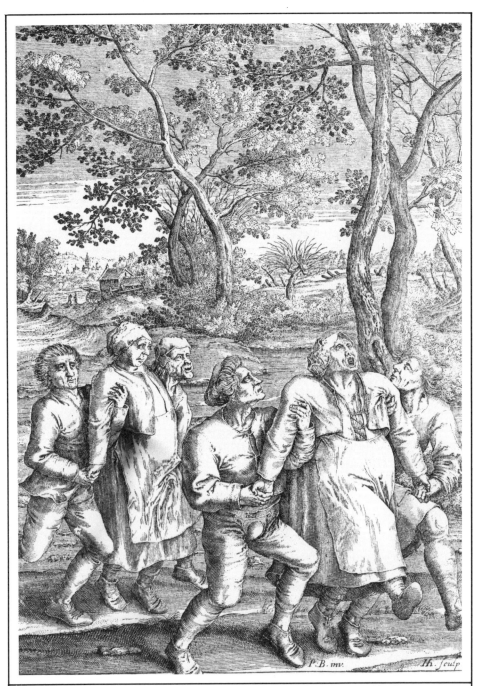

A 15th-century engraving depicts two victims of epilepsy. Modern medications can effectively treat seizure disorders but can also affect the body's reaction to other drugs such as alcohol.

CHAPTER 6

DRUGS AND CHRONIC DISEASE

Many children, teenagers, and young adults have chronic medical problems that require the use of medications on a daily or periodic basis. In order to keep these medical problems under control it is necessary for such individuals to understand both their diseases and their medications. Relatively common chronic problems in younger people (which may or may not be lifelong problems) include asthma, diabetes, and seizure disorders.

Asthma

Asthma is a disease of the respiratory system and is characterized by episodic severe constriction of the bronchial tree. This constriction makes breathing extremely difficult. The extra effort required to pull air into the lungs and then push it out produces the sound known as wheezing. Asthma occurs in people of all ages and can range from infrequent episodes of mild wheezing with colds or after vigorous exercise to frequent severe — even life-threatening — episodes that may or may not have an obvious cause.

Many children and adults are able to keep their asthma under control with a variety of medications. Some are pills or liquids, while others are inhaled mists.

As with any chronic illness, asthma should be treated by a physician. It is often necessary to adjust the amounts and types of medications taken as the patient grows or the symptoms change.

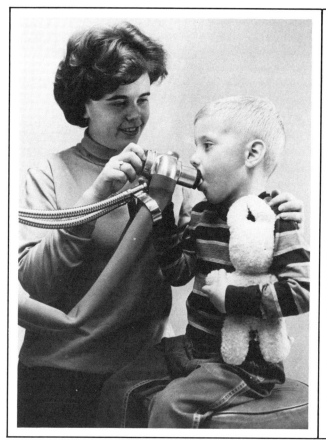

A mother assists her asthmatic son, who is using an apparatus that measures his lung capacity. Most asthma medications work by allowing the constricted muscles in the bronchial tree to relax.

The two most common classes of asthma medications — beta-adrenergic agents and theophylline — act by helping the constricted muscles in the bronchial tree relax.

The beta-adrenergic agents include epinephrine, isoetharine (Bronkosol), metaproterenol (Alupent), albuterol (Ventolin, Proventil), and others. Bronkosol, Ventolin, and Alupent are usually inhaled, but the last two are also available in oral form. Epinephrine is given as an injection for the treatment of severe asthma, life-threatening allergic reactions, and some other dangerous medical conditions.

Theophylline is a drug that shares many properties with caffeine. It comes in many different preparations that are taken orally, including Slo-bid and Theo-Dur. Some severe episodes are treated with a related drug called aminophylline, which is given intravenously. It is necessary to do blood tests periodically to make sure that people who use theophylline preparations are taking the right amount.

In most circumstances, flare-ups of wheezing can be controlled with the inhaled medications, either at home, in a doctor's office, or in a hospital emergency room. If treatment at home is unsuccessful it is important to call a doctor or go to a hospital as soon as possible.

Severe episodes, known as "status asthmaticus," usually require hospital admission for intravenous medications and frequent inhaler treatments. Occasionally, it is necessary to put a patient on a machine that breathes for him or her. The episode is rarely severe enough to be fatal.

All the common asthma medications are either true sympathomimetics or have side effects that involve activation of the sympathetic nervous system. The most common and annoying side effects are nervousness, restlessness, hand tremors, nausea, and vomiting. Overdose of an asthma medication can cause seizures, abnormal heart rhythms, and sometimes even death.

People who have asthma and are on medications must be aware of the interactions of these medications with other drugs, particularly the OTC sympathomimetics (see Chapter 5). For example, if someone who takes theophylline also takes an OTC cold preparation, significant sympathetic side effects are the likely result. In addition, erythromycin, a commonly used antibiotic, causes increased levels of theophylline in the blood and, if used in combination with theophylline, can be toxic.

OTC preparations of inhalable epinephrine are available (AsthmaNephrine, Bronkaid, Primatene, and others). This drug has strong side effects and should not be used casually.

Diabetes

Diabetes mellitus is a disorder of carbohydrate metabolism. People who have diabetes are unable to use sugars and starches — the breakdown products of carbohydrates in the diet — for energy. The ability to use carbohydrates effectively depends on the action of insulin, a hormone produced by special cells in the pancreas.

The basic source of energy for the human body is a sugar called glucose. As food is digested it is broken down to its simplest components, which are then absorbed from the intestines into the bloodstream and carried to various organs for further use. Carbohydrates are broken down to glucose.

In order for glucose to enter cells and supply energy, insulin must be present. The nervous system, the heart, exercising muscles, and the lens of the eye, however, can take up the minimum required amount of glucose without insulin.

Most people who develop diabetes as adults are able to produce insulin, but their bodies are unable to utilize it adequately. Children, teenagers, and young adults, on the other hand, develop what is known as insulin-dependent diabetes mellitus (IDDM). Their bodies are unable to produce enough insulin — often they cannot make any at all — so they depend on daily shots of insulin to live. Symptoms of IDDM include increased thirst, hunger, urination, and weight loss. It is often preceded by a viral illness.

As IDDM develops, glucose accumulates in the blood, reaching very high levels (hyperglycemia). The liver tries to supply the body with sufficient energy by forming more glucose, which cannot be used, and then by breaking down fats. One of the byproducts of the latter process is ketoacids, which also accumulate in the blood.

When hyperglycemia occurs, the kidneys try to bring the blood glucose level down to normal by filtering it out into the urine. Large amounts of urine are formed and excreted, and the body responds with increased thirst.

Because the liver uses all its energy stores to keep the body working, the body responds with increased hunger; despite the increased intake of food, however, weight is lost. Sometimes this condition is undetected for many weeks, and the person with IDDM becomes very ill from the combination of hyperglycemia and the accumulation of ketoacids in the blood, a condition known as diabetic ketoacidosis (DKA).

Some researchers believe that IDDM is simply an inherited disease. Others believe that only the tendency to develop the disease is inherited and that IDDM does not reveal itself unless the pancreas is damaged by the immune response to certain viruses.

Over time, diabetes can cause damage to the eyes, the kidneys, and other organs. Current research suggests that good control of blood sugar may help prevent severe problems later on.

Whatever the cause, IDDM is a lifelong disease that is controlled by the combination of a proper diet, regular exercise, and twice-daily injections of insulin. Most people use a combination of an immediate-acting and a long-acting insulin. The idea is to do with injections what the pancreas once did — supply the body with needed energy by facilitating the uptake of glucose from the blood into cells in all the organs and tissues. People with IDDM check the amount of glucose in their blood and urine to make sure they are using the right amount of insulin.

If too little insulin is used, the result is hyperglycemia, with return of the original symptoms of IDDM and the possibility of DKA.

If too much insulin is used, the blood glucose can go too low (hypoglycemia). Hypoglycemia can be life-threatening; the lack of sufficient glucose causes confusion and weakness and can lead to seizures and death. If discovered quickly, it can easily be treated by eating something high in

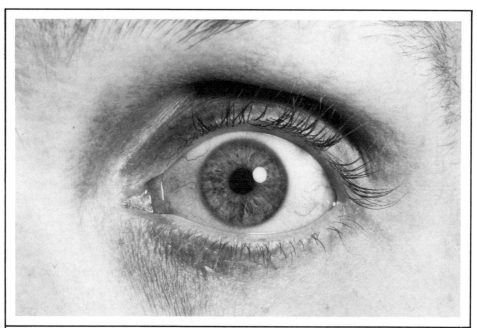

Diabetes is a dangerous disease that requires constant attention and medication. Among the many serious effects of this lifelong illness are blindness and other forms of eye damage.

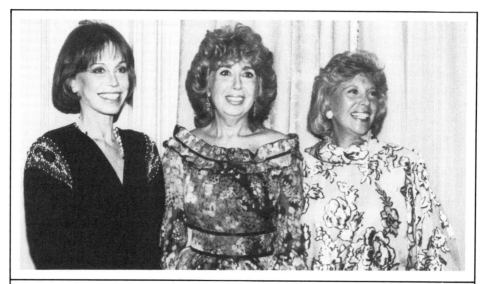

Mary Tyler Moore, Beverly Sills, and Dinah Shore pose at a fund-raising event for the Juvenile Diabetes Foundation. Research has still not determined the exact cause of this disease.

sugar like candy or orange juice; another treatment for hypoglycemia is an injection of *glucagon*, a hormone that releases stored glucose from the liver, raising the level of glucose in the blood.

IDDM is often a very frustrating disease for children and adults, because they must always be aware of how they feel, what they are eating, how much they are exercising, and how much insulin they need. Illness, very large or very small meals, and strenuous exercise all change the insulin requirement.

Many medications, including salicylates, antihypertensives, antidepressants, and sympathomimetics, alter the action of insulin. Many OTC drugs contain substantial amounts of sugar, but some preparations are made without sugar for people with IDDM.

It is important for an individual who has diabetes to let friends know what diabetes is and how it is treated. It is also important to recognize the signs of hyperglycemia and hypoglycemia, both of which can be very dangerous and must be treated as quickly as possible. It is wise to carry both extra insulin and a quick sugar source (usually candy) at all times to treat these problems early.

Seizure Disorders

A seizure is an abnormal discharge of electricity in the brain.

In the nervous system, electrical and chemical messages are passed in an orderly manner from nerve cell to nerve cell, directing normal body functions. During a seizure, electrical messages are out of control, like an electrical storm in the brain. Depending on which cells they affect, these scrambled messages may cause twitching of one or more parts of the body, strange sensations (an unusual taste, smell, or feeling), loss of consciousness, or a combination of these effects.

Seizures come in many varieties and have many different names. Often their cause is not known; these are called *idiopathic seizures*. Seizures are also classified according to how much of the body is affected and whether they involve loss of consciousness.

With proper medications most seizure disorders are well controlled and may even resolve over time in otherwise normal people. Many people with abnormal brain structures, either from birth or from later injuries, can have seizures that may be more difficult to control. On rare occasions, a seizure can signal the presence of a brain tumor or abnormal blood vessels in the brain; seizures can also occur during severe illnessess that may or may not directly affect the brain.

The most common types of seizures in young people are known as grand mal (big) and petit mal (little) seizures.

Grand mal, or generalized, seizures are the "fits" or "spells" that most people imagine when they think of epilepsy. This type of seizure may be preceded by an "aura," or warning sensation, often nausea, dizziness, or tingling. The person then loses consciousness and falls to the ground; the muscles then stiffen and the eyes roll back. This is usually followed by shaking of the arms and legs. The person may bite his or her tongue, drool, and urinate. The whole episode usually lasts only a few minutes. If a seizure does not stop in 20 to 30 minutes, it is necessary to stop it with intravenous medications.

Petit mal, or absence, seizures are brief episodes, generally lasting less than 10 seconds. They are characterized by "spacing out," or transient loss of consciousness, with staring. Occasionally they also include blinking of the eyes or smacking of the lips. They may occur dozens of times each day.

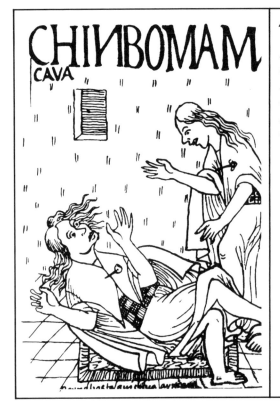

CHINBOMAM
CAVA

An Incan manuscript from the 16th century shows an epileptic suffering a seizure. In contemporary society many seizure disorders can be controlled with medication and may even resolve themselves over time.

The individual with this disorder is usually unaware of the episodes.

Children with petit mal seizures often come to medical attention because teachers, parents, and others believe they are daydreaming.

Grand mal seizures are usually treated with one or more of the following drugs: phenytoin (Dilantin), phenobarbital, and carbamazepine (Tegretol). In large doses all three depress the central nervous system and may cause lethargy and difficulty in walking and speaking. Overdoses of the drugs can interfere with the respiratory system and can be fatal.

Dilantin has been known to cause severe skin rashes. Phenobarbital sometimes causes hyperactivity rather than sedation and has been associated with learning disabilities. Tegretol, on occasion, causes blood disorders.

Petit mal seizures are usually treated with ethosuximide (Zarontin) or valproic acid (Depakene). In large doses these drugs also depress the central nervous system and therefore have some of the same side effects as the drugs used to treat grand mal seizures. Zarontin, like Tegretol, has been associated with blood disorders. Depakene has also been associated with liver disorders.

Because all these anticonvulsant (antiseizure) medications depress the nervous system, it is dangerous to take them in combination with other sedatives, particularly sleeping pills or alcohol.

Control of seizures is important both for medical and social reasons. It is embarrassing to have a seizure in a public place. It can also be dangerous to have a seizure while driving, riding a bicycle, swimming, or even crossing the street.

People who have seizure disorders can help themselves by taking their medication properly and making regular visits to a doctor. As with asthma medication, periodic blood tests are necessary to make sure that the right level of medication is present in the blood.

It is also important for people with seizure disorders to let someone know if they think they are going to have a seizure so medical attention can be obtained if needed.

If you are with someone who is having a seizure, the best thing to do is to make sure the person does not accidentally hurt himself or herself. If he or she seems to be having trouble breathing or if the seizure lasts more than a few minutes, call for help.

Conclusion

The human body is a delicate balance of systems and organs, maintained by nutrition, sleep, and a host of other factors. Disruption of any of the mechanisms that compose the infinitely complex organism that is the human body can disturb the balance necessary for good health. Drugs can be positive substances when they are used to restore the functions of the human body to normal. But when drugs are abused, they can themselves destroy bodily functions and cause short-term illness, chronic disease, and even death.

APPENDIX

State Agencies
for the Prevention and Treatment
of Drug Abuse

ALABAMA
Department of Mental Health
Division of Mental Illness and
  Substance Abuse Community
  Programs
200 Interstate Park Drive
P.O. Box 3710
Montgomery, AL 36193
(205) 271-9253

ALASKA
Department of Health and Social
  Services
Office of Alcoholism and Drug
  Abuse
Pouch H-05-F
Juneau, AK 99811
(907) 586-6201

ARIZONA
Department of Health Services
Division of Behavioral Health
  Services
Bureau of Community Services
Alcohol Abuse and Alcoholism
  Section
2500 East Van Buren
Phoenix, AZ 85008
(602) 255-1238

Department of Health Services
Division of Behavioral Health
  Services
Bureau of Community Services
Drug Abuse Section
2500 East Van Buren
Phoenix, AZ 85008
(602) 255-1240

ARKANSAS
Department of Human Services
Office of Alcohol and Drug Abuse
  Prevention
1515 West 7th Avenue
Suite 310
Little Rock, AR 72202
(501) 371-2603

CALIFORNIA
Department of Alcohol and Drug
  Abuse
111 Capitol Mall
Sacramento, CA 95814
(916) 445-1940

COLORADO
Department of Health
Alcohol and Drug Abuse Division
4210 East 11th Avenue
Denver, CO 80220
(303) 320-6137

CONNECTICUT
Alcohol and Drug Abuse
  Commission
999 Asylum Avenue
3rd Floor
Hartford, CT 06105
(203) 566-4145

DELAWARE
Division of Mental Health
Bureau of Alcoholism and Drug
  Abuse
1901 North Dupont Highway
Newcastle, DE 19720
(302) 421-6101

DISTRICT OF COLUMBIA
Department of Human Services
Office of Health Planning and
 Development
601 Indiana Avenue, NW
Suite 500
Washington, D.C. 20004
(202) 724-5641

FLORIDA
Department of Health and
 Rehabilitative Services
Alcoholic Rehabilitation Program
1317 Winewood Boulevard
Room 187A
Tallahassee, FL 32301
(904) 488-0396

Department of Health and
 Rehabilitative Services
Drug Abuse Program
1317 Winewood Boulevard
Building 6, Room 155
Tallahassee, FL 32301
(904) 488-0900

GEORGIA
Department of Human Resources
Division of Mental Health and
 Mental Retardation
Alcohol and Drug Section
618 Ponce De Leon Avenue, NE
Atlanta, GA 30365-2101
(404) 894-4785

HAWAII
Department of Health
Mental Health Division
Alcohol and Drug Abuse Branch
1250 Punch Bowl Street
P.O. Box 3378
Honolulu, HI 96801
(808) 548-4280

IDAHO
Department of Health and Welfare
Bureau of Preventive Medicine
Substance Abuse Section
450 West State
Boise, ID 83720
(208) 334-4368

ILLINOIS
Department of Mental Health and
 Developmental Disabilities
Division of Alcoholism
160 North La Salle Street
Room 1500
Chicago, IL 60601
(312) 793-2907

Illinois Dangerous Drugs
 Commission
300 North State Street
Suite 1500
Chicago, IL 60610
(312) 822-9860

INDIANA
Department of Mental Health
Division of Addiction Services
429 North Pennsylvania Street
Indianapolis, IN 46204
(317) 232-7816

IOWA
Department of Substance Abuse
505 5th Avenue
Insurance Exchange Building
Suite 202
Des Moines, IA 50319
(515) 281-3641

KANSAS
Department of Social Rehabilitation
Alcohol and Drug Abuse Services
2700 West 6th Street
Biddle Building
Topeka, KS 66606
(913) 296-3925

KENTUCKY
Cabinet for Human Resources
Department of Health Services
Substance Abuse Branch
275 East Main Street
Frankfort, KY 40601
(502) 564-2880

LOUISIANA
Department of Health and Human
    Resources
Office of Mental Health and
    Substance Abuse
655 North 5th Street
P.O. Box 4049
Baton Rouge, LA 70821
(504) 342-2565

MAINE
Department of Human Services
Office of Alcoholism and Drug
    Abuse Prevention
Bureau of Rehabilitation
32 Winthrop Street
Augusta, ME 04330
(207) 289-2781

MARYLAND
Alcoholism Control Administration
201 West Preston Street
Fourth Floor
Baltimore, MD 21201
(301) 383-2977

State Health Department
Drug Abuse Administration
201 West Preston Street
Baltimore, MD 21201
(301) 383-3312

MASSACHUSETTS
Department of Public Health
Division of Alcoholism
755 Boylston Street
Sixth Floor
Boston, MA 02116
(617) 727-1960

Department of Public Health
Division of Drug Rehabilitation
600 Washington Street
Boston, MA 02114
(617) 727-8617

MICHIGAN
Department of Public Health
Office of Substance Abuse Services
3500 North Logan Street
P.O. Box 30035
Lansing, MI 48909
(517) 373-8603

MINNESOTA
Department of Public Welfare
Chemical Dependency Program
    Division
Centennial Building
658 Cedar Street
4th Floor
Saint Paul, MN 55155
(612) 296-4614

MISSISSIPPI
Department of Mental Health
Division of Alcohol and Drug Abuse
1102 Robert E. Lee Building
Jackson, MS 39201
(601) 359-1297

MISSOURI
Department of Mental Health
Division of Alcoholism and Drug
    Abuse
2002 Missouri Boulevard
P.O. Box 687
Jefferson City, MO 65102
(314) 751-4942

MONTANA
Department of Institutions
Alcohol and Drug Abuse Division
1539 11th Avenue
Helena, MT 59620
(406) 449-2827

NEBRASKA
Department of Public Institutions
Division of Alcoholism and Drug
Abuse
801 West Van Dorn Street
P.O. Box 94728
Lincoln, NB 68509
(402) 471-2851, Ext. 415

NEVADA
Department of Human Resources
Bureau of Alcohol and Drug Abuse
505 East King Street
Carson City, NV 89710
(702) 885-4790

NEW HAMPSHIRE
Department of Health and Welfare
Office of Alcohol and Drug Abuse
   Prevention
Hazen Drive
Health and Welfare Building
Concord, NH 03301
(603) 271-4627

NEW JERSEY
Department of Health
Division of Alcoholism
129 East Hanover Street CN 362
Trenton, NJ 08625
(609) 292-8949

Department of Health
Division of Narcotic and Drug
   Abuse Control
129 East Hanover Street CN 362
Trenton, NJ 08625
(609) 292-8949

NEW MEXICO
Health and Environment Department
Behavioral Services Division
Substance Abuse Bureau
725 Saint Michaels Drive
P.O. Box 968
Santa Fe, NM 87503
(505) 984-0020, Ext. 304

NEW YORK
Division of Alcoholism and Alcohol
   Abuse
194 Washington Avenue
Albany, NY 12210
(518) 474-5417

Division of Substance Abuse
   Services
Executive Park South
Box 8200
Albany, NY 12203
(518) 457-7629

NORTH CAROLINA
Department of Human Resources
Division of Mental Health, Mental
   Retardation and Substance Abuse
   Services
Alcohol and Drug Abuse Services
325 North Salisbury Street
Albemarle Building
Raleigh, NC 27611
(919) 733-4670

NORTH DAKOTA
Department of Human Services
Division of Alcoholism and Drug
   Abuse
State Capitol Building
Bismarck, ND 58505
(701) 224-2767

OHIO
Department of Health
Division of Alcoholism
246 North High Street
P.O. Box 118
Columbus, OH 43216
(614) 466-3543

Department of Mental Health
Bureau of Drug Abuse
65 South Front Street
Columbus, OH 43215
(614) 466-9023

OKLAHOMA
Department of Mental Health
Alcohol and Drug Programs
4545 North Lincoln Boulevard
Suite 100 East Terrace
P.O. Box 53277
Oklahoma City, OK 73152
(405) 521-0044

OREGON
Department of Human Resources
Mental Health Division
Office of Programs for Alcohol and
  Drug Problems
2575 Bittern Street, NE
Salem, OR 97310
(503) 378-2163

PENNSYLVANIA
Department of Health
Office of Drug and Alcohol
  Programs
Commonwealth and Forster Avenues
Health and Welfare Building
P.O. Box 90
Harrisburg, PA 17108
(717) 787-9857

RHODE ISLAND
Department of Mental Health,
  Mental Retardation and Hospitals
Division of Substance Abuse
Substance Abuse Administration
  Building
Cranston, RI 02920
(401) 464-2091

SOUTH CAROLINA
Commission on Alcohol and Drug
  Abuse
3700 Forest Drive
Columbia, SC 29204
(803) 758-2521

SOUTH DAKOTA
Department of Health
Division of Alcohol and Drug Abuse
523 East Capitol, Joe Foss Building
Pierre, SD 57501
(605) 773-4806

TENNESSEE
Department of Mental Health and
  Mental Retardation
Alcohol and Drug Abuse Services
505 Deaderick Street
James K. Polk Building,
  Fourth Floor
Nashville, TN 37219
(615) 741-1921

TEXAS
Commission on Alcoholism
809 Sam Houston State Office
  Building
Austin, TX 78701
(512) 475-2577
Department of Community Affairs
Drug Abuse Prevention Division
2015 South Interstate Highway 35
P.O. Box 13166
Austin, TX 78711
(512) 443-4100

UTAH
Department of Social Services
Division of Alcoholism and Drugs
150 West North Temple
Suite 350
P.O. Box 2500
Salt Lake City, UT 84110
(801) 533-6532

VERMONT
Agency of Human Services
Department of Social and
  Rehabilitation Services
Alcohol and Drug Abuse Division
103 South Main Street
Waterbury, VT 05676
(802) 241-2170

VIRGINIA
Department of Mental Health and
　Mental Retardation
Division of Substance Abuse
109 Governor Street
P.O. Box 1797
Richmond, VA 23214
(804) 786-5313

WASHINGTON
Department of Social and Health
　Service
Bureau of Alcohol and Substance
　Abuse
Office Building—44 W
Olympia, WA 98504
(206) 753-5866

WEST VIRGINIA
Department of Health
Office of Behavioral Health Services
Division on Alcoholism and Drug
　Abuse
1800 Washington Street East
Building 3 Room 451
Charleston, WV 25305
(304) 348-2276

WISCONSIN
Department of Health and Social
　Services
Division of Community Services
Bureau of Community Programs
Alcohol and Other Drug Abuse
　Program Office
1 West Wilson Street
P.O. Box 7851
Madison, WI 53707
(608) 266-2717

WYOMING
Alcohol and Drug Abuse Programs
Hathaway Building
Cheyenne, WY 82002
(307) 777-7115, Ext. 7118

GUAM
Mental Health & Substance Abuse
　Agency
P.O. Box 20999
Guam 96921

PUERTO RICO
Department of Addiction Control
　Services
Alcohol Abuse Programs
P.O. Box B-Y Rio Piedras Station
Rio Piedras, PR 00928
(809) 763-5014

Department of Addiction Control
　Services
Drug Abuse Programs
P.O. Box B-Y Rio Piedras Station
Rio Piedras, PR 00928
(809) 764-8140

VIRGIN ISLANDS
Division of Mental Health,
　Alcoholism & Drug Dependency
　Services
P.O. Box 7329
Saint Thomas, Virgin Islands 00801
(809) 774-7265

AMERICAN SAMOA
LBJ Tropical Medical Center
Department of Mental Health Clinic
Pago Pago, American Samoa 96799

TRUST TERRITORIES
Director of Health Services
Office of the High Commissioner
Saipan, Trust Territories 96950

Further Readings

Danaher, B.G. and Lichenstein, E. *Become an Ex-Smoker*. Englewood Cliffs, New Jersey: Prentice-Hall, 1978.

Fielding, Jonathan E. "Smoking: Health Effects and Control: Part I," in *New England Journal of Medicine*, vol. 313, no. 8, p. 491: August 22, 1985.

Harms, Ernest, ed. *Drugs and Youth: The Challenge of Today*. New York: Pergamon Press, 1973.

Heath, Robert G. *Marijuana & the Brain*. Rockville, Maryland: American Council on Marijuana, 1981.

Lindesmith, A.R. *Addiction and Opiates*. Chicago: Aldine Publishing, 1968.

Mosher, Beverly A. *The Health Effects of Caffeine*. New York: The American Council on Science and Health, 1981.

Glossary

acute of sudden onset and exhibited in severe symptoms occurring over a short period of time

addiction a condition caused by repeated drug use, characterized by a compulsive urge to continue using the drug, a tendency to increase the dosage, and physiological and/or psychological dependence

alcoholism alcohol abuse causing deterioration in health and social relations

alkaloid one of many organic substances containing nitrogen that strongly affect body functions; drugs such as morphine and cocaine are alkaloids

asthma respiratory distress which occurs when the muscles of the bronchial tree constrict

autonomic nervous system the part of the nervous system that is concerned with the control of involuntary bodily functions

cancer a group of diseases characterized by a disordered growth of cells that may form tumors, invade local tissues, or spread to distant sites

carcinogens substances that are thought to cause cancer

central nervous system the brain and the spinal cord

chronic a long-term problem that may wax and wane, but is always present

chronic obstructive lung disease a group of diseases that impede the lung's normal functioning; these diseases include emphysema and chronic bronchitis and can be progressively debilitating

delirium tremens (DTs) the withdrawal syndrome a chronic alcoholic suffers when his alcohol supply is cut off; symptoms include anxiety, tremors, sweating, and hallucinations, and sometimes death

epidemiology the study of various epidemic diseases that includes attempts to prevent or control their spread in the general population

fetal alcohol syndrome a condition in which a mother's heavy drinking during pregnancy produces a specific set of physical and mental handicaps in her developing fetus; the symptoms include growth deficiency, a particular pattern of facial deformities, brain and spinal cord defects, and varying degrees of malfunctions in major organs

heart attack sudden chest pains that may extend to the arms and throat of the victim; can be fatal

hemoglobin an iron-rich structure in the red blood cells that carries oxygen from the lung to body tissues

hormone a product of a living cell that is carried by the bloodstream to other cells, which it stimulates by chemical action

hyperglycemia an abnormally high blood-sugar level, a condition commonly found in people suffering from diabetes mellitus

hypoglycemia an abnormally low blood-sugar level that causes muscular weakness, mental disorientation, sweating and poor coordination

infertility failure of a man or woman's reproductive system to function adequately

insulin the protein hormone that controls the amount of sugar (glucose) in the bloodstream

insulin-dependent diabetes mellitus (IDDM) a disorder in which insulin production is either insufficient or absent, causing impaired carbohydrate metabolism and necessitating the use of insulin injections

metabolism the combination of anabolism (synthesizing large, complex molecules from small ones) and catabolism (the breakdown of large molecules into small ones), which affects nutrition and use of energy in the body

myocardial infarction death of a portion of heart muscle caused by an interruption of its blood supply; a victim consequently suffers a heart attack

neurotransmitter a chemical released by neurons that transmits nerve impulses across a synapse

nicotine a poisonous alkaloid and component of tobacco believed to be responsible for the addictive properties of cigarettes

overdose a large quantity of a drug taken accidentally or on purpose, which causes temporary or permanent damage to the body and may be fatal

over-the-counter medications (OTCs) legal drugs that are available without a doctor's prescription

passive smoking inhaling the "second-hand smoke" exhaled by smokers, or the smoke that comes from the burning end of a cigarette

physical dependence adaption of the body to the presence of a drug such that its absence produces withdrawal symptoms

psychological dependence a condition in which the drug user craves a drug to maintain a sense of well-being and feels discomfort when deprived of it

seizures abnormal bursts of electrical activity in the brain that are manifested as short periods of disordered movement, behavior or sensations, with or without loss of consciousness

side effects desirable or undesirable effects a drug may have on an individual that arise in addition to the substance's anticipated effects

stimulants substances that temporarily increase functional abilities of certain body organs and cause a sense of increased well-being and alertness; side effects may include loss of appetite, irritability and gastric distress

sympathomimetics drugs that imitate the neurotransmitters norepinephrine and epinephrine, causing activation of the sympathetic nervous system (a part of the autonomic nervous system)

tolerance a decrease of susceptibility to the effects of a drug due to its continued administration, resulting in the user's need to increase the drug dosage in order to achieve the effects experienced previously

withdrawal the physiological and psychological effects of discontinued use of a drug

Picture Credits

Index

Laurel Shader, M.D., is currently a Resident in Pediatrics at Yale-New Haven Hospital. She earned an A.B. in English and American Literature at Brown University and her M.D. degree at Tufts University School of Medicine.

Jon Zonderman is an author and journalist who specializes in the coverage of scientific and technological issues. He also teaches journalism at Columbia University Graduate School of Journalism and Fordham University. He holds an A.B. in American Studies from Trinity College and an M.S. from the Columbia School of Journalism.

Solomon H. Snyder, M.D., is Distinguished Service Professor of Neuroscience, Pharmacology and Psychiatry at The Johns Hopkins University School of Medicine. He has served as president of the Society for Neuroscience and in 1978 received the Albert Lasker Award in Medical Research. He has authored *Uses of Marijuana, Madness and the Brain, The Troubled Mind, Biological Aspects of Mental Disorder,* and edited *Perspective in Neuropharmacology: A Tribute to Julius Axelrod.* Professor Snyder was a research associate with Dr. Axelrod at the National Institutes of Health.

Barry L. Jacobs, Ph.D., is currently a professor in the program of neuroscience at Princeton University. Professor Jacobs is author of *Serotonin Neurotransmission and Behavior* and *Hallucinogens: Neurochemical, Behavioral and Clinical Perspectives.* He has written many journal articles in the field of neuroscience and contributed numerous chapters to books on behavior and brain science. He has been a member of several panels of the National Institute of Mental Health.

Joann Ellison Rodgers, M.S. (Columbia), became Deputy Director of Public Affairs and Director of Media Relations for the Johns Hopkins Medical Institutions in Baltimore, Maryland, in 1984 after 18 years as an award-winning science journalist and widely read columnist for the Hearst newspapers.